THE PINK SALT MORNING RITUAL FOR WOMEN OVER 40

The 5-Minute Morning Ritual to Melt Belly Bloat, Boost Energy, Crush Cravings, and Support Natural Weight Loss During Menopause and Perimenopause

CHRISTINA ARDIANI

Ediciones Ardiani

CONTENTS

Disclaimer   vii

Introduction   ix

1. UNDERSTANDING THE OVER-40 BODY: WHY THINGS FEEL DIFFERENT NOW   1
Why Things Feel Different Now   1
Why Everything Feels Different Now   2
The Metabolism Myth   3
Hormones in Plain English   4
Why Stress Changes Everything   6
Sleep, Hunger, and Energy   7
Muscle, Movement, and Daily Burn   8
Water Retention Versus Real Fat Gain   9
Why Restrictive Diets Often Backfire   11
What Your Body Needs Now   12

2. THE PINK SALT TRUTH: WHAT HELPS, WHAT DOESN'T, AND WHY THIS RITUAL MATTERS   14
There is something deeply human about the search for a simple solution.   14
Why Pink Salt Became So Popular   15
What Pink Salt Actually Is   16
What Pink Salt Can Realistically Help With   18
What Pink Salt Cannot Do   19
Why the Ritual Still Matters   20
Sodium, Bloating, and Smart Use   22
Who Should Be Cautious   23
How to Choose a Good Pink Salt Product   23
The Bigger Picture   24

3. THE 5-MINUTE MORNING RESET RITUAL   26
Think about the last time you had a genuinely good morning.   26
Why Mornings Matter More Than You Think   27
The Power of a 5-Minute Ritual   28
The Core Pink Salt Morning Ritual   29
Optional Ritual Variations   30
Add a Body Reset in Motion   31
The Mindset Minute   32

How to Make the Ritual Automatic   33
What If You Miss a Day?   34
Your First 21 Days   35

4. BEAT BELLY BLOAT AND FEEL LIGHTER FAST   38
There is a particular kind of frustration that arrives in the evening.   38
Why Bloating Feels So Defeating   39
Fat Versus Bloat: Understanding the Difference   40
Why Bloating Often Increases After 40   41
Common Food and Lifestyle Triggers   42
Hidden Sodium and Puffiness   44
Gut-Friendly Daily Habits   44
Evening Habits for a Flatter Morning   46
Your 7-Day Debloat Reset   47
Progress Beyond a Flat Stomach   48

5. CRUSH CRAVINGS, BOOST ENERGY, AND STOP EMOTIONAL EATING   49
It usually happens at the same time every day.   49
Why Cravings Feel Stronger Now   50
Willpower Is Not the Real Problem   51
The Afternoon Energy Crash   52
Emotional Eating in Real Life   53
Build Meals That Reduce Cravings   55
Quick Energy Boosters That Actually Help   56
The Craving Rescue Plan   57
How to Bounce Back After a Bad Day   58
Becoming a Woman Who Trusts Herself Again   59

6. LET'S TALK ABOUT SOMETHING THAT ALMOST NO ONE TALKS ABOUT HONESTLY.   61
Let's talk   61

7. THE 21-DAY PINK SALT RESET PLAN   73
You have spent five chapters building understanding.   73
Why 21 Days Matters   74
How to Use This Plan   75
Week One: Reduce Bloat and Build Momentum   75
Week Two: Stabilize Energy and Reduce Cravings   77
Week Three: Build Lasting Weight-Loss Habits   78
What to Track Beyond the Scale   80
If Progress Feels Slow   81

What Happens After Day 21   82

Your Fresh Start Begins Now   83

Conclusion: Your New Chapter Starts Now   85

Disclaimer

The content in this book is provided for educational and informational purposes only. While every effort has been made to ensure accuracy, the publisher and author make no guarantees regarding the completeness or reliability of the information presented.

The publisher and author disclaim any liability for decisions made or actions taken based on the information contained in this book.

DISCLAIMER

Medical Disclaimer

The information contained in *The Pink Salt Morning Ritual for Women Over 40* is intended for educational and informational purposes only. It is not medical advice, and it is not a substitute for professional medical guidance, diagnosis, or treatment.

Every woman's body and health history is unique. Before making any changes to your diet, lifestyle, or daily habits, please consult a qualified healthcare professional — especially if you have an existing health condition, take prescription medications, or have any concerns about your personal health.

If something you read in these pages raises questions, bring them to a licensed professional you trust. That is always the right step.

Nothing in this book is intended to diagnose, treat, cure, or prevent any medical condition. Individual results will vary. Never disregard or delay seeking professional medical advice because of something you have read here.

Christina Ardiani

INTRODUCTION

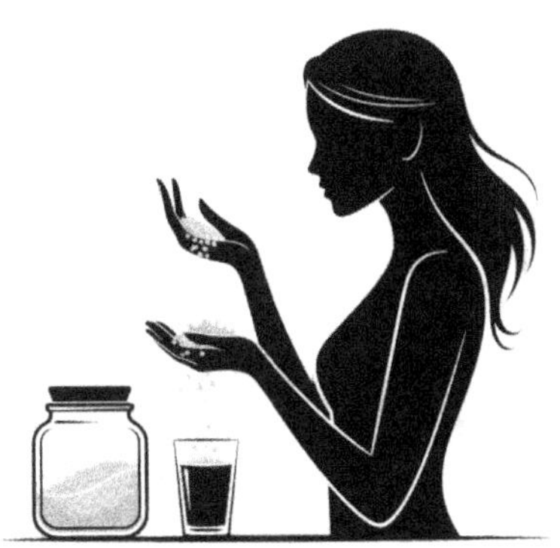

THERE IS A PARTICULAR KIND OF FRUSTRATION THAT ONLY WOMEN WHO HAVE LIVED IT WILL TRULY UNDERSTAND.

It is not the dramatic frustration of a sudden crisis. It is quieter than that, and in many ways more exhausting. It is the frustration of waking up one morning and realizing that the body you have known your entire adult life has quietly started playing by a different set of rules, rules nobody bothered to explain to you, and rules that seem to change just when you think you have figured them out.

Maybe it started gradually. A little more puffiness around your midsection after dinner. Jeans that fit perfectly last spring suddenly feeling uncomfortably tight by mid-afternoon, even though you have not changed a single thing about what you eat. A heaviness that settles into your lower belly by evening like a slow tide coming in, leaving you unbuttoning the top button in private and wondering what on earth is happening to you.

Or maybe the energy was the first thing you noticed. That easy, reliable vitality you once had, the kind that carried you through busy days, workouts, social plans, and late nights without much complaint, slowly started feeling harder to access. Not impossible. Just... dimmer. Like a light you keep turning up, only to find the bulb has quietly lost some of its wattage.

And the cravings. Oh, the cravings. Sweet things you never used to care much about. Salt. Carbs. That inexplicable urge at three in the afternoon or ten at night that feels less like hunger and more like desperation, a craving that is almost emotional, almost physical, almost impossible to ignore no matter how much willpower you throw at it.

If any of this sounds familiar, I want you to take a slow breath right now, because I need you to hear something important before we go any further:
This is not your fault.
Not a single bit of it.

You did not become less disciplined. You did not suddenly lose your motivation or your self-control. You did not fail at being healthy. What happened is that your body entered a profound biological transition, one that touches nearly every system you have — your hormones, your metabolism, your gut, your sleep, your mood, your energy regulation — and it did so without a roadmap, without much warning, and in a culture that is still embarrassingly underprepared to support women through it.

Perimenopause and menopause are not minor events. They are not simply the end of a monthly cycle. They are a full hormonal recalibration that can take years, unfolding differently in every woman's body, reshaping the landscape of how you feel, how you look, how you digest food, how you sleep, and how you experience yourself from the inside out.

Estrogen, progesterone, cortisol, insulin — these are not just words in a biology textbook. They are the invisible orchestrators of your energy, your mood, your hunger signals, your belly fat distribution, your bloating, and your relationship with food. And when they begin to shift, as they naturally do in your forties and fifties, everything you thought you knew about how your body works can start to feel unreliable.

The diet that kept you lean in your thirties no longer moves the needle. The exercise routine that used to energize you now leaves you depleted. The glass of wine that once relaxed you now disrupts your sleep and leaves you puffy the next morning. The healthy meal you ate for dinner somehow translates to a bloated, uncomfortable belly by bedtime.

It is maddening. And it is real. And it deserves to be taken seriously.

Here is where so many women go wrong — and I say this with enormous compassion, because the pressure to find a solution is completely understandable.

When the body stops responding the way it used to, the natural instinct is to try harder. To restrict more. To cut another food group. To push through tougher workouts. To download another app and start tracking every bite again. To white-knuckle through another Monday, another detox, another round of elimination eating, searching for the specific thing that broke and the specific fix that will put it right.

And sometimes, for a brief window, something works. The scale moves. The bloat backs off a little. You feel a flicker of hope. But then, almost inevitably, the progress stalls. The cravings come back with force. The energy dips again. Life gets busy and the rigid plan becomes impossible to sustain, and suddenly you are back at the beginning — except now you are carrying a little more self-doubt than before, a little more quiet belief that maybe your body is just broken, or maybe you just do not have what it takes anymore.

That story ends here. Right now, on this page.

The problem was never your willpower. The problem was the approach — strategies built for younger hormonal environments being applied to a body that has fundamentally changed. Strict restriction raises cortisol, which in a perimenopausal body is the last thing you want, because elevated cortisol actively encourages belly fat storage and worsens sleep, which worsens cravings, which makes restriction harder, which raises cortisol further. It is a cycle designed for failure, not because you are failing, but because the strategy itself is working against your biology.

What your body needs now is not more force. It is more support.

We live in an age of wellness miracles, and nowhere is that more visible than in the world of women's health online. Every week brings a new superfood, a new supplement stack, a new morning drink that promises to melt belly fat while you sleep, reset your hormones with one teaspoon, and solve every symptom of menopause by next Tuesday.

The viral promises are seductive, and understandably so. When you are exhausted and frustrated and looking for relief, hope is a powerful thing — even when it arrives dressed up in bold claims and glowing testimonials.

Pink Himalayan salt has had its own moment in this landscape, and the stories you may have encountered online range from the genuinely interesting to the wildly overstated. Yes, there is real science behind hydration, electrolyte balance, and mineral support. Yes, a thoughtful morning hydration ritual can be a meaningful tool for reducing bloat, improving energy, and anchoring a healthier daily routine. These are not empty claims.

But no, a pinch of pink salt dissolved in water is not going to single-handedly transform your hormones, eliminate your belly fat, or undo years of metabolic shifts in a matter of days. Anyone who tells you otherwise is selling you a fantasy, and you deserve better than fantasies.

What you deserve is the truth — offered warmly, practically, and with genuine respect for your intelligence and your experience.

This book is built on that foundation.

So what is the Pink Salt Reset, really?

It is not a miracle cure dressed up in pretty packaging. It is a framework for rebuilding your mornings, your hydration habits, your relationship with food, and your overall daily rhythm in a way that genuinely supports a peri-menopausal and menopausal body.

The pink salt morning ritual is where it begins — a simple, intentional act of waking up and giving your body what it is often desperately asking for: hydration, trace minerals, and a gentle signal that the day is starting with care rather than chaos. It is a small thing, and small things matter enormously, not because they are magic, but because they are the kind of consistent, manageable action that actually gets done, day after day, in a real and busy life.

From that morning anchor, the reset expands outward. It includes practical guidance on eating in a way that works with your shifting hormones rather than against them — not a strict diet, not a list of forbidden foods, but a nourishing approach that supports steady energy, reduces the inflammation and water retention that drive so much of that uncomfortable bloat, and helps your body find its natural hunger and fullness signals again.

It includes simple strategies for supporting your sleep, managing the kind of chronic low-grade stress that is silently driving belly fat and cravings in millions of women over forty, and building a daily rhythm that feels sustainable and kind rather than punishing and temporary.

It includes honest conversation about what is happening in your body and why — explained in plain, human language that empowers you rather than overwhelms you. Because when you understand what is actually going on, the symptoms that once felt random and frightening start to make sense. And when things make sense, they become workable.

This is not about perfection. It is about progress that lasts.

Here is what I want you to imagine, just for a moment.

Imagine waking up tomorrow morning and having a ritual waiting for you — something small, gentle, and entirely your own. A moment of quiet intention before the day begins. Warm water, a small pinch of pink salt, maybe a squeeze of lemon. A breath. A choice to start differently.

Imagine that over the coming days, you begin to notice your mornings feeling a little cleaner. The heavy, foggy feeling that used to sit on your shoulders before your first coffee starts lifting a little earlier. Your belly feels a little less tight, a little less uncomfortable. You begin to make small shifts to your eating rhythm that do not feel like deprivation, but like nourishment, and your body begins responding with less inflammation, more steadiness, fewer of those desperate mid-afternoon crashes.

Imagine your jeans fitting more comfortably not because you starved yourself but because you started working with your body's actual needs. Imagine standing in front of the mirror and feeling, not shame or frustration, but something softer — a kind of quiet reconnection with yourself, a sense that you are no longer at war.

Imagine feeling like you again. Not a younger version, not a perfect version — just you, in your own skin, with your own energy, feeling capable and comfortable and genuinely well.

That is what this book is designed to help you build. Not overnight. Not with a single magic ingredient. But steadily, realistically, and in a way that fits inside your actual life.

As you move through these pages, I want to invite you to release any expectation that this has to be approached perfectly. There is no gold star waiting for the woman who reads every chapter in order and implements every strategy simultaneously. Progress in a perimenopause or menopause context is rarely linear, and this journey is not designed with rigidity in mind.

Read at your own pace. Try one thing at a time. Notice what resonates and begin there. Some chapters will feel immediately relevant to where you are right now; others may become more meaningful later. There is no wrong way to move through this material, as long as you keep moving.

What matters most is not speed. It is not perfection. It is not doing everything at once. What matters is that you begin — gently, compassionately, with the understanding that your body is not your enemy, and that the changes you are experiencing are not a sentence you are serving, but a transition you are navigating, with more tools and more support than you may have had before.

You picked up this book for a reason. Something in you is ready — ready for something that actually works, that respects your body's current reality, that offers hope without hype and solutions without shame.

I am so glad you are here.

Let's begin.

UNDERSTANDING THE OVER-40 BODY: WHY THINGS FEEL DIFFERENT NOW

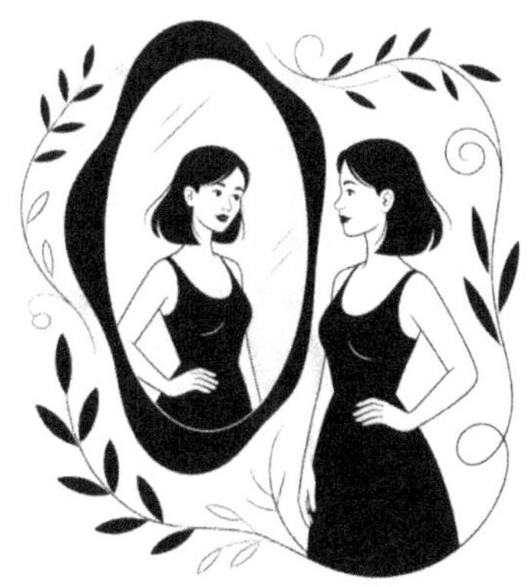

WHY THINGS FEEL DIFFERENT NOW

There is a moment that many women describe in almost identical terms, regardless of where they live, what they do, or how they have spent their adult lives taking care of themselves.

It usually happens somewhere between the ages of forty and fifty. Sometimes it arrives quietly, like a slow dimming. Sometimes it feels more sudden, as though a switch was thrown overnight. But the experience is remarkably consistent: you look in the mirror, or you step off the scale, or you pull on a pair of jeans that fit perfectly six months ago, and something registers that you cannot quite explain. Something has shifted. Not just physically, though the physical changes are real. Something deeper. A sense that the reliable relationship you once had with your own body — the unspoken agreement between you and your metabolism, your energy, your hunger — has quietly been renegotiated without your input.

If that resonates with you, you are not imagining things. You are not being dramatic. And you are most certainly not alone.

What you are experiencing is the result of genuine, significant biological change — change that is normal, natural, and shared by every woman who lives long enough to move through midlife. But normal does not mean easy, and natural does not mean painless or simple to navigate. The fact that these changes are universal does not make them any less disorienting when they arrive in your particular body, in your particular life, and begin rearranging things you thought were settled.

This chapter is here to help you understand what is actually happening — not in the language of medical textbooks or complicated research papers, but in plain, honest terms that make the picture clearer and, more importantly, make the path forward feel workable. Because here is the truth that this entire book is built upon: your body is not broken. It has not turned against you. It is not punishing you for your choices or your age. It is changing, and change — even frustrating, uncomfortable, bewildering change — is something that can be understood, supported, and worked with.

Let's start at the beginning.

WHY EVERYTHING FEELS DIFFERENT NOW

For most of your twenties and thirties, your body operated on a set of relatively predictable principles. Eat a little less, move a little more, and the scale would eventually cooperate. Skip the bread for a week, drink more water, go for a few runs, and things would shift. Not always quickly, not always dramatically, but the system was essentially responsive. You pushed the right levers and the body responded. It was not always easy, but it made sense.

After forty, and particularly as you approach and move through perimenopause, that responsiveness begins to change. The levers that used to work reliably start producing different results, or no results at all. You cut your calories and feel exhausted but do not lose weight. You exercise faithfully and your belly stays exactly where it is. You eat what you have always eaten and somehow gain several pounds in a matter of months. You skip dinner and wake up more bloated than when you went to bed. Nothing adds up in the way it used to, and the absence of logic is one of the most frustrating parts of the whole experience.

This is not a failure of effort or willpower. It is a failure of the old framework to account for what is actually happening in your body.

The changes that begin in your forties are widespread and interconnected. Your hormones are shifting — not just the reproductive ones, but the hormones that regulate your appetite, your stress response, your sleep architecture, your blood sugar, and your fat storage patterns. Your muscle mass, if you have not been actively working to maintain it, may be quietly declining, which changes the rate at which your body burns energy at rest. Your gut microbiome, which has enormous influence over digestion, bloating, nutrient absorption, and even mood, is sensitive to hormonal fluctuation and can shift in ways that produce new symptoms. Your sleep quality may be deteriorating, which has cascading effects on hunger hormones, energy, mood, and metabolism.

None of these changes happen in isolation. They are deeply woven together, each one influencing the others in a complex web that can be difficult to untangle — and even more difficult to address with the blunt instruments of simple calorie restriction and extra cardio.

Understanding this interconnection is the first and most important step. Not because knowledge alone will solve anything, but because it replaces the false narrative of personal failure with an accurate picture of biological reality. You are not doing something wrong. Your body has changed in ways that require a different approach. That is a problem that can be solved. It just requires different tools.

THE METABOLISM MYTH

Ask most women over forty why they are gaining weight, and the answer comes quickly and with a kind of resigned certainty: my metabolism has slowed down. It is one of the most widely accepted explanations in women's wellness, repeated so often that it has become almost unquestioned.

And there is truth in it — but it is a partial truth, and the parts that get left out are the parts that actually give you power.

Yes, metabolic rate does tend to decline with age. Research consistently shows that the number of calories your body burns at rest decreases as you get older. But the magnitude of this decline is often significantly overstated in popular culture, and — more importantly — metabolism is not a fixed, immutable thing. It is a dynamic process influenced by factors you have far more control over than you might have been led to believe.

The single largest driver of metabolic rate, outside of basic organ function, is muscle tissue. Muscle is what researchers call metabolically active tissue, meaning it burns calories simply by existing, even when you are sitting completely still. The more muscle you carry, the more energy your body requires to sustain itself around the clock. And beginning in your thirties, the average person begins to lose muscle mass at a gradual but meaningful rate — a process called sarcopenia — that accelerates without deliberate effort to counter it.

This is why two women of the same age and weight can have very different metabolic rates, and why the woman who has maintained or built muscle through consistent movement will find weight management considerably more manageable than the woman who has relied on cardio alone or, worse, on chronic undereating, which actively breaks down muscle tissue to use for fuel.

But metabolism is also influenced by sleep, and chronic sleep deprivation — which becomes far more common for many women during perimenopause — measurably reduces metabolic efficiency and increases the hormones that drive fat storage. It is influenced by chronic stress, which elevates cortisol and creates conditions in which your body preferentially stores fat around the abdomen. It is influenced by how consistently you eat and how well you nourish yourself, because severely restricting calories for extended periods sends your body into an adaptive state where it deliberately conserves energy by slowing metabolic processes down.

So yes, metabolism changes. But the story of why it changes, and what you can do about it, is far richer and more empowering than the simple phrase "my metabolism has slowed" suggests. You are not at the mercy of an inexorably declining engine. You are navigating a system that responds — intelligently, if sometimes frustratingly — to the conditions you create for it.

That is good news. Because conditions can be changed.

HORMONES IN PLAIN ENGLISH

If there is one topic that comes up in nearly every conversation about women's health over forty, it is hormones. And for good reason — the hormonal shifts of perimenopause and menopause are genuinely significant, genuinely far-reaching, and genuinely responsible for many of the changes that feel most disorienting during this time.

But hormones are also a topic that gets explained poorly, either in impenetrable clinical language that leaves most people more confused than when they started, or in oversimplified terms that make hormones sound like a single dial that has simply been turned down. The reality is more nuanced than either extreme, and understanding the key players — even in broad strokes — can completely change how you interpret what your body is doing.

Let's talk about the ones that matter most for the changes you are likely experiencing.

Estrogen is the hormone most people associate with femininity and reproduction, but its role in the body extends far beyond those domains. Estrogen influences bone density, cardiovascular health, skin elasticity, mood regulation, and cognitive function. It also plays a significant role in how your body distributes and stores fat. When estrogen levels are balanced and sufficient, fat tends to be distributed more evenly across the body, with a preference for the hips and thighs. As estrogen declines in perimenopause and menopause, this distribution pattern changes, and the body begins storing more fat centrally — around the abdomen and waist. This is the biological explanation for the belly that appears to arrive from nowhere, even in women who have not changed their eating habits at all.

Estrogen also influences insulin sensitivity, which affects how efficiently your body processes and uses carbohydrates for energy. As estrogen declines, many women become somewhat less insulin sensitive, meaning the same amount of carbohydrates can produce a larger blood sugar response — which in turn can contribute to increased fat storage, more intense sugar cravings, and the kind of energy spikes and crashes that leave you reaching for something sweet by mid-afternoon.

Progesterone works in balance with estrogen, and when that balance is disrupted — as it often is during perimenopause, when progesterone typically declines before estrogen does — the effects can be significant. Progesterone has a naturally calming, sleep-supporting effect on the body. It promotes GABA activity in the brain, which is associated with relaxation and restorative sleep. When progesterone drops, sleep often becomes lighter and more disrupted, anxiety can increase, and the nervous system can feel persistently activated in a way that makes it much harder to wind down in the evenings. Progesterone also has a mild natural diuretic effect, meaning that when it declines, some women notice increased water retention and bloating that can feel both physically uncomfortable and deeply disheartening when they see it reflected on the scale.

Cortisol is your primary stress hormone, produced by the adrenal glands in response to both physical and psychological stress. In appropriate amounts and at appropriate times, cortisol is genuinely useful — it mobilizes energy, sharpens alertness, and helps you respond to demands and challenges. The problem arises when cortisol is elevated chronically, which is increasingly common in the lives of women navigating busy careers, caregiving responsibilities, financial pressures, relationship demands, and the additional physiological stress of hormonal transition itself.

Chronically elevated cortisol does several things that are particularly problematic for women over forty. It promotes the storage of visceral fat — the deep abdominal fat that accumulates around organs and contributes to that stubborn belly fullness that resists conventional dieting. It interferes with sleep quality, creating a vicious cycle in which poor sleep elevates cortisol further, which worsens sleep, and so on. It disrupts the normal function of thyroid hormones, which play a central role in metabolic rate. And it directly counteracts the effects of progesterone, meaning that high chronic stress can intensify the symptoms of hormonal imbalance significantly.

For busy women over forty, cortisol is often the overlooked piece of the puzzle. You may be eating reasonably well and exercising consistently, but if your nervous system is locked in a state of chronic activation — if you are perpetually rushing, worrying, overwhelmed, and under-rested — your body will prioritize survival and fat storage over weight loss, regardless of what the rest of your approach looks like.

Insulin is the hormone responsible for transporting glucose from the bloodstream into cells, where it can be used for energy. When insulin function is optimal, this process is smooth and efficient. When cells become resistant to insulin's signal — a state called insulin resistance — the body produces more and more insulin in an attempt to do the same job, and the excess insulin creates conditions that favor fat storage, increase hunger and cravings, and make sustained energy very difficult to achieve.

Insulin resistance becomes more common after forty for several reasons: declining estrogen, increased cortisol, reduced muscle mass, disrupted sleep, and the natural tendency for fat cells around the abdomen to be particularly resistant to insulin's effects. It is a key driver of the energy crashes, carbohydrate cravings, and persistent belly fat that so many women experience during this time — and it is also highly responsive to lifestyle intervention, which means it is one of the most actionable pieces of the hormonal puzzle.

Understanding these four hormones does not require a degree in endocrinology. What matters is simply this: the hormonal environment of your forties and fifties is genuinely different from what it was before, and that environment shapes how your body stores fat, how it regulates hunger, how it manages energy, and how it responds to the approaches you take to care for it. Working with that environment — rather than fighting against it with strategies designed for a different hormonal context — is the key to making real, lasting progress.

WHY STRESS CHANGES EVERYTHING

It would be easy to address stress in a single paragraph, acknowledge it as important, and move on to the more tangible topics of food and exercise. Most wellness books do exactly that.

But stress deserves more than a passing mention, because for women in their forties and fifties, it is often the central force that is quietly sabotaging every other effort — and it is the one factor that is most consistently underestimated or completely ignored.

Think about the average day in the life of a woman at this stage of life. She may be managing a demanding career while simultaneously navigating the particular pressures of midlife — aging parents who need increasing support, children who are moving through their own complex transitions, relationships that require attention and energy, financial responsibilities that feel heavier than ever. She may be experiencing the psychological weight of watching her body change in ways she cannot fully control, carrying grief for the version of herself that felt effortless and capable in ways that now feel distant. And she is doing all of this in a body that is producing less of the hormones that once served as a natural buffer against stress.

This is not a small thing. This is an enormous physiological load.

When the body perceives stress — whether that stress is a genuine emergency or the relentless low-grade pressure of an overfull life — it activates the same basic survival system. The hypothalamic-pituitary-adrenal axis, which is your body's central stress-response network, signals the adrenal glands to release cortisol and adrenaline. Heart rate increases, digestion slows, and the body mobilizes energy from fat and muscle to prepare for action.

This is extraordinarily useful if you need to run from a predator. It is profoundly unhelpful if it is happening in a low-level, persistent way as you respond to emails, worry about money, care for aging parents, and lie awake at three in the morning running through your to-do list.

When cortisol is chronically elevated, digestion is compromised — contributing directly to the bloating and digestive discomfort that so many women over forty experience, often without any obvious dietary explanation. Appetite regulation is disrupted, with cortisol specifically increasing cravings for dense, calorie-rich foods — the sweet and salty things that provide rapid energy and activate the brain's reward pathways in ways that feel, momentarily, like relief. Sleep quality deteriorates, because elevated cortisol in the evenings directly interferes with the hormonal cascade that should be winding your nervous system down for rest.

And the body's fat distribution shifts. Visceral fat — the fat that accumulates deep in the abdominal cavity — is particularly sensitive to cortisol, and it also happens to be the fat that is most visible as a thickening around the midsection, the belly that sits differently than it used to, the waistline that seems to have disappeared.

Stress eating is not a character flaw. It is a physiological response. When cortisol spikes, so do hunger signals, and the foods that feel most compelling during stress are precisely the foods that activate the calm-and-reward centers of the brain. Understanding this does not make it easier to eat a salad when your nervous system is screaming for a chocolate bar, but it does remove the layer of shame and self-judgment that compounds the problem — because shame is itself a stressor that elevates cortisol further.

The most important implication of all of this is that stress management is not a luxury or a nice-to-have. For women over forty, it is a non-negotiable component of any approach to weight, energy, and hormonal health. Not because you need to be perfectly zen or eliminate difficulty from your life — which is neither possible nor realistic — but because supporting your nervous system's ability to recover from stress, even in small ways throughout the day, changes the biochemical environment in which everything else you do takes place.

SLEEP, HUNGER, AND ENERGY

If you are sleeping poorly, everything else becomes harder. This is not motivational rhetoric — it is physiology.

Sleep is when your body performs a remarkable amount of its most important maintenance work. Hormones are regulated, cells are repaired, memories are consolidated, inflammatory processes are resolved, and the brain clears metabolic waste that accumulates during waking hours. When sleep is disrupted, shortened, or architecturally altered — as it frequently is during perimenopause and menopause, thanks to the combined effects of declining progesterone, night sweats, and elevated evening cortisol — the downstream consequences are extensive and immediate.

Among the most impactful effects of poor sleep are changes in two key appetite-regulating hormones: ghrelin and leptin. Ghrelin is the hormone that signals hunger, telling your brain it is time to eat. Leptin is the hormone that signals satiety, telling your brain you have had enough. Sleep deprivation consistently raises ghrelin and suppresses leptin — which means that after a poor night's sleep, you are biochemically hungrier, less able to feel full, and significantly more likely to crave high-calorie, high-carbohydrate foods. This is not a lack of willpower. It is hormonal instruction.

Research has consistently shown that even a single night of poor sleep can increase caloric intake the following day by several hundred calories, with most of the increase coming from snacks and from foods that are dense in sugar and fat. Multiply that effect across weeks or months of disrupted sleep — which is the reality for many women during perimenopause — and the impact on weight and energy is significant and measurable.

Beyond hunger, poor sleep depletes motivation and cognitive clarity in ways that make every healthy choice feel harder. The version of you who is well-rested can plan ahead, make thoughtful decisions about food, and find genuine enjoyment in movement. The version of you who is exhausted operates on a shortened decision-making runway, reaching for convenience and comfort because the prefrontal cortex — the part of the brain responsible for planning and impulse control — is genuinely impaired by sleep deprivation in measurable, documented ways.

This is why, in this reset, sleep is treated as a pillar — not an afterthought. The woman who sleeps well is hormonally, neurologically, and energetically better positioned for every single other aspect of this journey. Supporting your sleep is not indulgent. For women navigating midlife hormonal change, it may be the single most powerful thing you can do.

MUSCLE, MOVEMENT, AND DAILY BURN

There is a persistent myth in women's fitness culture that the path to a leaner, lighter body runs through hours of intense cardio — classes, long runs, cycling sessions that leave you drenched and depleted. Sweat harder, burn more, lose weight. It is a simple equation that has been sold to women for decades.

The problem is that this equation becomes less accurate as you age, and can actively work against you after forty.

Here is what matters more than almost anything else when it comes to supporting your metabolism, managing your weight, and maintaining your physical vitality as a woman in midlife: muscle.

Muscle tissue is metabolically expensive. It requires energy to maintain, even at rest, and the more of it you carry, the higher your resting metabolic rate. This means that two women of identical weight who carry different amounts of muscle will burn different numbers of calories over the course of every single day — not just during exercise, but while sitting, sleeping, working, and doing everything else that makes up a life.

After forty, and accelerating after menopause, women are at significant risk of losing muscle mass if they do not actively work to preserve or build it. This happens for several reasons: declining estrogen reduces the anabolic (muscle-building) signaling that was previously present, protein synthesis becomes less efficient with age, and activity levels often decline as life gets busier and more sedentary. The result is a gradual reshaping of body composition — less muscle, more fat, a slower metabolism — that explains a great deal of the weight gain that women experience in midlife even without significant changes to their eating habits.

The solution is not extreme. You do not need to become a competitive athlete or spend two hours daily in the gym. Resistance training — lifting weights, using resistance bands, doing bodyweight exercises like squats, lunges, and push-ups — done two to three times per week with enough challenge to create a stimulus for muscle development, is genuinely transformative for women over forty. It is one of the most evidence-supported interventions for maintaining metabolic health, improving body composition, supporting bone density, reducing the risk of injury, and improving quality of life through midlife and beyond.

Daily movement matters too — not as a calorie-burning strategy, but as a way of maintaining insulin sensitivity, supporting circulation, reducing stress hormones, improving sleep quality, and giving your body the consistent physical activity signal it evolved to receive. Walking is genuinely powerful. Not because it burns enormous calories, but because it does so many other things well, and because it is sustainable and accessible in a way that intense exercise often is not.

The goal here is not punishment or performance. It is sustainability, consistency, and choosing forms of movement that you can genuinely imagine yourself doing next year, and the year after that — because the benefits of movement are cumulative, and the woman who walks thirty minutes a day for a decade will almost always be healthier than the one who crushes intense workouts for three months and then burns out entirely.

WATER RETENTION VERSUS REAL FAT GAIN

This section may be one of the most practically relieving things you read in this entire book.

A significant portion of the weight fluctuation, the morning puffiness, the belly that feels bigger after some days than others, and the discouraging number you sometimes see on the scale is not fat. It is water — held in tissues as a result of hormonal fluctuation, dietary patterns, stress, disrupted digestion, and the body's constant effort to maintain fluid balance in a rapidly shifting internal environment.

This is not a comforting fiction. It is real physiology.

Estrogen and progesterone both influence how the body regulates water retention. During the hormonal fluctuations of perimenopause, water balance can shift dramatically from day to day. A drop in progesterone, in particular, removes a natural diuretic effect and can cause noticeable fluid retention, especially around the abdomen and in the face and hands. Salt intake, processed foods, alcohol, and inflammatory foods can worsen this effect considerably — not because they are causing fat gain, but because they are triggering the body to hold onto water in amounts that translate to visible physical changes and real differences on the scale.

The digestive component is equally significant. Bloating — the tightness, distension, and discomfort that many women over forty experience regularly — is often driven by gut bacteria imbalances, slowed digestion, food sensitivities that may have developed or intensified in midlife, and the effects of stress and cortisol on gastrointestinal function. A bloated belly is not a fat belly, even though it can feel indistinguishable from one. And crucially, the solutions for bloat — better hydration, gut-supporting foods, stress reduction, gentler eating habits — are different from the solutions for fat loss.

Understanding the difference matters enormously, both practically and emotionally. When you wake up two pounds heavier than you were yesterday, despite doing everything right, and you know that it is almost certainly a combination of water retention and digestive factors rather than actual fat accumulated overnight, you can respond with curiosity and targeted support rather than despair and restriction. You can ask what your body might need — more water, a lighter day of eating, some movement to get things moving, a stress-reducing evening routine — instead of concluding that everything is hopeless and you might as well give up.

The scale measures everything — muscle, fat, water, the food in your digestive tract, the clothes you are wearing. It is a crude instrument for tracking body composition, and treating its daily fluctuations as meaningful data will drive you quietly mad. This reset will help you build a much healthier relationship with your body and its signals, one that is based on how you feel, how your clothes fit, and how you are consistently caring for yourself — rather than a number that can change by three pounds depending on how much water you drank the day before.

WHY RESTRICTIVE DIETS OFTEN BACKFIRE

You have probably been here before. The decision arrives on a Sunday evening, or a Monday morning, or after a particularly uncomfortable day when nothing in your wardrobe feels right. Enough is enough. Starting tomorrow, things will be different. Calories will be cut. Certain foods will be eliminated. The discipline will be fierce, the commitment total.

And for a while, it works. Weight comes off, sometimes quite quickly in those first one to two weeks, which provides enough positive reinforcement to keep going. But then something shifts. The cravings become more intense rather than less. The energy dips to a point that makes daily function genuinely difficult. Sleep worsens. Irritability rises. Social situations become fraught. The restrictive approach starts requiring more and more willpower to maintain, and willpower is a finite resource that eventually runs out — especially when your body is being deprived of the fuel, nourishment, and pleasure it genuinely needs.

And then comes the rebound. Often fast, often painful, often resulting in more weight gained back than was lost, accompanied by a fresh layer of shame and the conviction that you simply lack the self-control required to succeed.

This cycle is not a character flaw. It is biology.

When you significantly restrict calories, your body interprets this as a famine signal and responds accordingly — slowing metabolic rate, increasing hunger hormones, reducing the energy available for non-essential functions, and creating a neurological preoccupation with food that is almost impossible to override through sheer determination. This response evolved to keep humans alive in environments where food scarcity was a real survival threat. It is a brilliantly designed protective mechanism that has no idea it is operating during a voluntary diet rather than an actual famine.

For women over forty, this dynamic is intensified by the hormonal context. Elevated cortisol from stress and restriction further slows metabolism and promotes fat storage. Disrupted sleep from hunger and blood sugar instability worsens cravings. Reduced intake of protein and essential nutrients accelerates the muscle loss that was already being driven by hormonal change. The body is not being uncooperative or stubborn. It is doing exactly what it is designed to do — and doing it more efficiently than ever, in a body that has become increasingly skilled at conservation.

The all-or-nothing pattern — perfect compliance followed by total abandonment — is particularly common among women who have spent years cycling through restrictive approaches, and it is emotionally exhausting in ways that compound the physical challenges. Every restart carries the weight of previous attempts. Every slip feels not like a minor deviation but like a total failure that negates everything. The emotional toll is real, and it matters.

What works better — significantly better, and particularly so for women navigating midlife hormonal change — is a gentler, more consistent, more nourishing approach. One that supports your body with enough food, enough protein, enough variety to preserve muscle and fuel energy. One that reduces, rather than intensifies, the stress load on your already stretched nervous system. One that builds sustainable habits gradually, values consistency over perfection, and treats the occasional imperfect day as exactly that — an imperfect day, not a catastrophic failure requiring complete restart.

WHAT YOUR BODY NEEDS NOW

Here is the hopeful truth, and it is a real one: your body is incredibly responsive to care.

Not punishment. Not extreme measures. Care.

The changes that are happening in your forties and fifties are real and significant, but they are not the end of the story. They are a transition — and transitions, by definition, are movements between one state and another. The state you are moving toward does not have to be one of resignation and difficulty. With the right understanding and the right tools, it can be one of genuine vitality, comfort, and confidence.

What your body needs now is different from what it needed at twenty-five or thirty-five, and recognizing that is not defeat — it is intelligence. It means you can stop applying the wrong solutions to the right problem. It means you can meet your body where it actually is, rather than where you wish it still was.

Hydration is more important than you likely realize. As estrogen declines, the body's ability to retain water in tissues changes, and many women in perimenopause and menopause are walking around in a state of chronic mild dehydration without knowing it. Dehydration worsens bloating, impairs digestion, reduces energy, intensifies cravings, and clouds cognitive function. Drinking enough water — and drinking it in a way that your cells can actually use, supported by trace minerals — is one of the simplest and most impactful things you can do for your daily wellbeing.

Nourishment, in the form of protein-rich, nutrient-dense eating that supports muscle maintenance and stable blood sugar, is far more effective than restriction. Your body needs building blocks — adequate protein, healthy fats, fiber-rich vegetables, complex carbohydrates in proportions that work for your current insulin sensitivity — not deprivation. Feeding yourself well is not in conflict with weight management. For women over forty, it is the foundation of it.

Better daily rhythms — consistent sleep and wake times, eating patterns that work with your body's natural circadian biology, morning routines that anchor calm and intention rather than reactive rushing — create the hormonal environment in which your body functions at its best. These are not luxuries. They are biological necessities for a body navigating significant hormonal transition.

Movement that builds and preserves muscle, supports daily energy expenditure, reduces stress hormones, and feels enjoyable enough to sustain over time. Not punishment, not obsessive exercise, but consistent, varied, progressive movement that honors what your body can do.

And support for your nervous system — real, practical strategies for interrupting the chronic stress cycles that are quietly driving so many of the symptoms that feel most out of control. Sleep support. Breathing practices. Reducing the unnecessary load where you can. Learning to recognize the difference between pushing through and burning out.

This is what the Pink Salt Reset is built on. The morning ritual that opens this journey is not a magic solution — it is a signal. A daily act of intention that says: today, I am going to start by giving my body something it needs. And from that small, consistent beginning, everything else becomes a little easier to build.

You are not starting over. You are starting smarter.

The chapters ahead will walk you through each piece of this in practical, actionable detail — the food strategies that work with your hormones rather than against them, the hydration and mineral support that can transform how you feel within days, the movement approach that protects your metabolism and your long-term health, and the daily rituals that make all of it feel sustainable rather than exhausting.

Your body brought you here. It is asking for something different, and you are wise enough to listen.

Let's keep going.

2

THE PINK SALT TRUTH: WHAT HELPS, WHAT DOESN'T, AND WHY THIS RITUAL MATTERS

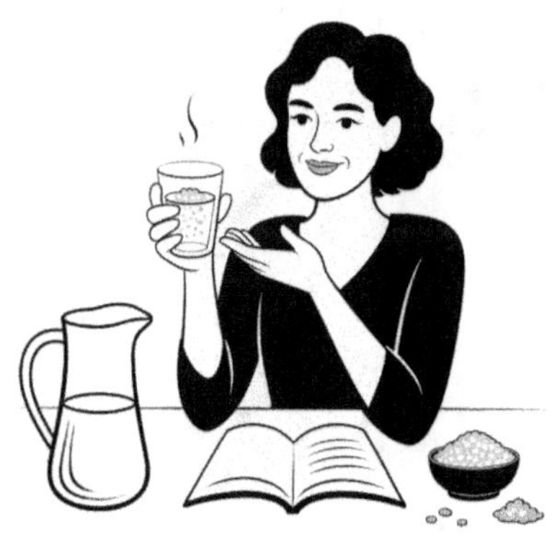

THERE IS SOMETHING DEEPLY HUMAN ABOUT THE SEARCH FOR A SIMPLE SOLUTION.

When life is complicated — when your body is changing in ways that feel out of your control, when every diet you have tried has eventually let you down, when you are exhausted and bloated and quietly desperate for something that actually works — the appeal of a single, beautiful, natural remedy is almost irresistible. Something you can hold in your hand. Something with a name that sounds ancient and pure. Something that promises to cut through all the confusion and give you back the feeling of being well.

Pink Himalayan salt arrived in the wellness world at exactly the right moment to fill that role. And it arrived with considerable style.

The photographs alone are enough to understand the appeal — that warm, rosy, crystalline mineral sitting in a wooden bowl, dissolved into a glass of clear water catching the morning light, arranged beside a lemon and a few sprigs of something green. It looks like wellness. It looks intentional and natural and somehow both ancient and aspirational at the same time. On social media, it became the visual shorthand for a particular kind of woman: the woman who wakes up before her family, who moves through her morning with calm and purpose, who takes care of herself as a daily act of devotion rather than an occasional crisis response.

And then the claims began to multiply. Detoxifies the body. Balances hormones. Burns belly fat. Boosts metabolism. Cures bloating overnight. Restores mineral deficiencies. Transforms your energy in days.

If you have spent any time online researching wellness solutions for women over forty, you have almost certainly encountered versions of these promises — some of them dressed in the language of science, some accompanied by before-and-after photographs, many offered by people selling products alongside their testimonials. And if you are anything like most women who come to this book, you have had some version of the same internal experience: a flash of hope, followed by a familiar wariness, followed by the question that is increasingly difficult to silence: is this real, or is this just another thing that is going to disappoint me?

This chapter is the honest answer to that question. All of it — what pink salt actually is, what it can genuinely help with, what it cannot do, and why the ritual built around it still matters more than you might expect.

WHY PINK SALT BECAME SO POPULAR

To understand why pink Himalayan salt captured the imagination of the wellness world, it helps to understand the broader landscape it arrived in.

The early decades of the twenty-first century brought a significant cultural shift in how people — and particularly women — think about health and well-being. The era of purely clinical, pharmaceutical, expert-dictated health guidance began giving way to something more personal, more natural, more connected to ancient wisdom and simple living. People started reading ingredient labels. They started asking where their food came from. They started questioning the assumption that synthetic, processed, manufactured solutions were inherently superior to natural ones.

Alongside this shift came the rise of social media as a primary vehicle for health information and inspiration. Instagram, Pinterest, YouTube, and eventually TikTok created platforms where wellness culture could spread visually and virally, and where the aesthetic of health became as important as the substance of it. Beautiful food, beautiful rituals, beautiful bodies engaged in beautiful morning routines — these images circulated with extraordinary speed and reach, building aspirational frameworks for how health could look and feel.

Pink Himalayan salt fit this aesthetic perfectly. It is genuinely beautiful. Its warm pink color is visually distinctive in a world of white table salt. Its origins — ancient sea beds in the Himalayan region, untouched by modern pollution, harvested by hand and minimally processed — tell a compelling story that resonates with people who are increasingly skeptical of industrially processed food. It feels natural in a way that a white crystalline powder in a blue cardboard cylinder does not.

The appeal was also practical in its simplicity. Here was something you could add to a glass of water. Something that cost very little. Something that required no special equipment, no prescription, no complicated preparation. In a wellness landscape that often demands significant investment of time, money, and expertise, the pink salt morning water ritual was remarkably accessible.

And then the community formed around it. Women shared their experiences — real ones, genuine ones, accounts of feeling better, sleeping more soundly, noticing less bloating, having more energy. These experiences were real, even when the reasons behind them were more complex than a simple salt supplement. The ritual worked for many people, not necessarily because pink salt is a miracle mineral, but because it was the anchor of a broader morning routine that supported healthier choices throughout the day. More on that shortly.

What spread fastest, as tends to happen in wellness culture, were the most dramatic claims. The nuanced, accurate version — this is a pleasant mineral salt that supports hydration habits and makes a lovely anchor for a morning wellness routine — does not go viral. The version that promises to melt belly fat and balance hormones does. And so the gap widened between what pink Himalayan salt can actually do and what many people have come to believe it does, and millions of women have arrived at their own disappointing crossroads between expectation and reality.

You deserve a more honest starting point. And that starts with understanding exactly what pink salt is.

WHAT PINK SALT ACTUALLY IS

Pink Himalayan salt is a rock salt mined primarily from the Khewra Salt Mine in the Punjab region of Pakistan — not from the Himalayas themselves, though its marketing name has stuck firmly enough that correction feels almost pedantic at this point. It is one of the largest and oldest salt mines in the world, and the deposits it contains are ancient — formed hundreds of millions of years ago from the evaporation of prehistoric seas, long before the kinds of industrial pollution that characterize modern environments existed.

Its distinctive pink color comes from trace amounts of iron oxide — rust, essentially — along with small quantities of other minerals that give different crystals slightly different hues, ranging from pale blush to deep rose to occasional white or gray. The color is genuine, not added, and it is one of the few things about pink salt marketing that is entirely accurate.

Chemically, pink Himalayan salt is predominantly sodium chloride — the same compound that makes up regular table salt, which is also sodium chloride. This is the fundamental fact that sits at the center of any honest conversation about pink salt: at its core, it is salt. The differences are real but modest.

Table salt, as most people know it, is heavily refined. The refining process strips out most naturally occurring minerals and leaves an extremely pure sodium chloride product. Many commercial table salts also contain added iodine — a practice that began in the 1920s in response to widespread iodine deficiency and the resulting thyroid disorders — along with anti-caking agents to keep the crystals from clumping.

Pink Himalayan salt is less refined and contains a broader mineral profile as a result. Alongside sodium and chloride, it contains small amounts of potassium, magnesium, calcium, iron, and a range of other trace minerals. Studies have identified over eighty different mineral compounds in Himalayan salt, which is a genuinely impressive number and has been the source of considerable enthusiasm in wellness circles.

Here is where it is important to stay grounded in proportion: the quantities of these additional minerals are very small. A typical serving of pink salt — one quarter teaspoon dissolved in a glass of water, which is roughly what the morning ritual involves — contains trace mineral amounts that are real but modest relative to what your body obtains from a varied diet. The magnesium in a quarter teaspoon of pink salt, for example, is a fraction of what you would get from a small handful of almonds, a cup of leafy greens, or a piece of dark chocolate. The potassium is far exceeded by a single banana.

This does not make those minerals meaningless. Trace minerals matter, and in a world where many people are not eating as varied and nutrient-dense a diet as they should be, every additional mineral source has some value. But it does mean that the mineral content of pink salt, while genuinely present and genuinely broader than refined table salt, is not the dramatic nutritional intervention it is sometimes portrayed as.

Pink salt also contains slightly less sodium per teaspoon than table salt, simply because its larger, less uniform crystals pack together less densely — meaning you get slightly less sodium in the same measured volume. This difference is real but unlikely to be meaningful in most practical contexts.

What pink Himalayan salt is, then, is a minimally processed, aesthetically pleasing, pleasantly flavored salt with a genuine trace mineral profile and a somewhat lower sodium density than refined table salt. It is a modest upgrade from standard table salt in some respects, a lateral move in others, and a significant improvement in exactly none of the dramatic ways it is often promoted.

That is the honest assessment. And now we can talk about what it can actually help with.

WHAT PINK SALT CAN REALISTICALLY HELP WITH

The most meaningful thing that a pinch of pink salt dissolved in morning water can do is support hydration — and that, it turns out, is not a small thing at all.

Hydration is one of the most fundamentally important factors in how you feel on any given day, and it is also one of the most widely neglected. Research consistently shows that a large proportion of adults are chronically mildly dehydrated — not dramatically, not in ways that feel like thirst, but in ways that show up as fatigue, difficulty concentrating, sluggish digestion, headaches, and yes, bloating. The digestive system requires adequate hydration to function smoothly, and when it does not have enough, gut motility slows, gas accumulates, and that tight, uncomfortable fullness around the abdomen can worsen considerably.

For women over forty, the hydration picture becomes more complicated. Estrogen plays a role in the body's fluid regulation mechanisms, and as estrogen declines, some of those mechanisms become less efficient. The sensation of thirst can become less reliable as a signal — meaning you may not feel particularly thirsty even when your cellular hydration is below optimal. Many women in perimenopause and menopause are, without realizing it, under-hydrating in ways that contribute to fatigue, brain fog, and digestive discomfort.

Drinking a glass of water first thing in the morning addresses this directly. After seven to nine hours of fasting and breathing through the night, your body wakes up in a state of relative dehydration, and rehydrating before caffeine, before food, before the demands of the day begin, is one of the most straightforwardly beneficial things you can do for your morning energy and digestion.

The addition of a small amount of pink salt to this morning water has a genuine rationale behind it. Sodium is an electrolyte — a mineral that carries an electrical charge in fluid and plays a central role in fluid balance, nerve function, and the transport of water into cells. A very small amount of sodium in your morning water can support the body's ability to actually absorb and use that water at a cellular level, rather than having it pass through quickly before it can be properly utilized. This is the principle behind oral rehydration solutions and electrolyte drinks used in medical and athletic contexts, applied in a much gentler, more modest form.

This effect is real, and it is one of the reasons some people genuinely notice a difference in how they feel after incorporating the morning water ritual — more awake, less sluggish, better digested — compared to plain water alone. It is not magic. It is basic hydration physiology, and pink salt happens to be a pleasant and natural way to access it.

Beyond the direct hydration effect, the morning pink salt ritual supports wellbeing in a way that is perhaps even more significant: it creates a moment of intention at the start of the day.

This matters more than it might sound. The act of preparing your morning water, making a considered choice to begin your day with something nourishing before the reactive demands of the day begin, signals something to your brain about the kind of day you are about to have. It is a small act of self-care that activates the identity of someone who takes care of themselves. And that identity activation, as we will discuss shortly, tends to ripple outward into better choices throughout the rest of the day.

The ritual also supports consistency, which is the single most underrated factor in any wellness approach. The best strategy in the world, practiced inconsistently, will produce far less meaningful change than a modest strategy practiced reliably, day after day. A morning ritual that is simple enough to do every single day — regardless of how busy or tired or unmotivated you feel — is worth more than a complex protocol you can only manage when circumstances are perfect.

WHAT PINK SALT CANNOT DO

This is the section that some books leave out, and its absence is part of why so many women end up disappointed, confused, and questioning their own efforts rather than questioning the exaggerated claims they were sold.

Pink salt dissolved in water will not burn your belly fat. Not a little, not indirectly, not over time through some complex metabolic pathway. The sodium chloride and trace minerals in a quarter teaspoon of dissolved salt do not interact with adipose tissue, do not stimulate lipolysis, do not alter the hormonal environment in ways that promote fat loss, and do not create a calorie deficit. Fat loss requires a sustained energy deficit — consistently burning more energy than you consume over time — and no morning drink, however natural and mineral-rich, creates that condition on its own.

It will not balance your hormones. Hormonal health is influenced by many interconnected factors — nutrition, body weight, sleep quality, stress levels, physical activity, liver function, thyroid health, and the underlying biological timetable of perimenopause and menopause. These are complex systems that respond to sustained, consistent lifestyle support. They are not meaningfully altered by a trace mineral supplement delivered in a glass of water.

It will not detoxify your body. Your body already has a sophisticated detoxification system — primarily your liver and kidneys — that operates continuously and remarkably efficiently when you support it through adequate hydration, good nutrition, and avoiding excessive toxic loads. You do not need a special substance to activate this system, and pink salt is not a detoxifier by any meaningful biochemical definition of the term.

It will not compensate for poor sleep. Sleep deprivation produces a cascade of hormonal and metabolic consequences — elevated cortisol, disrupted hunger signaling, impaired insulin sensitivity, reduced energy expenditure — that cannot be corrected by any mineral or beverage. If your sleep is significantly disrupted, the morning ritual will offer some support, but addressing sleep directly remains essential.

It will not override a diet that is significantly out of alignment with your body's needs. If the rest of your eating is high in processed foods, refined sugars, excess sodium from packaged products, and insufficient protein and fiber, a glass of pink salt water will not meaningfully change the nutritional picture. The morning ritual matters most as the first act of a broader pattern, not as a standalone corrective.

Understanding this is not discouraging. It is clarifying. Because the women who are most disappointed by wellness products and rituals are almost always the women who were given unrealistic expectations in the first place — who believed, and were sometimes explicitly told, that a single simple intervention would solve a complex problem. When that single intervention inevitably fails to deliver a transformation on its own, the disappointment is profound and the self-blame is unfair.

Pink salt is a genuinely useful, enjoyable, and meaningful part of a morning wellness ritual. It is not a miracle. And you are strong enough to work with the truth.

WHY THE RITUAL STILL MATTERS

Here is the thing about rituals: they work, and they work in ways that go far deeper than the physical properties of any single ingredient they involve.

Human beings are profoundly ritualistic creatures. We have always organized our days, our transitions, and our major life events around meaningful repeated actions — practices that signal something important to the conscious and subconscious mind alike. Morning rituals, in particular, have been shown in behavioral research to have a meaningful impact on how the rest of the day unfolds, not because of magic, but because of psychology.

When you begin your day with an intentional action — something you chose, something that represents care for yourself, something that connects you to a vision of the person you want to be — you activate what researchers call behavioral activation and identity priming. You are not just drinking a glass of water. You are taking an action that is consistent with the identity of someone who takes care of their body, who begins the day with purpose rather than reactive chaos, who values their own wellbeing enough to act on it first thing in the morning.

And identity, it turns out, is one of the most powerful drivers of sustained behavior change. The woman who thinks of herself as someone who takes care of her health will make hundreds of small decisions throughout the day differently from the woman who does not hold that identity — not through conscious deliberation, but through the invisible filter of who she believes she is. A simple morning ritual, practiced consistently, gradually shifts that identity. You begin to see yourself as the kind of person who does this. And the kind of person who does this also tends to make better choices about what she eats for breakfast, whether she gets outside for a walk, how she manages her response to stress.

Rituals also reduce decision fatigue, which is a genuine and measurable phenomenon. The cognitive resources you have available for decision-making in any given day are not unlimited, and they are depleted by every choice you make — including the small, seemingly trivial ones. Having a settled morning ritual means there is one significant category of morning decisions that requires no deliberation: you simply do the thing you always do. This preservation of cognitive resources can make better decisions easier throughout the rest of the day, simply because you are not starting from a depleted baseline.

There is also the momentum effect. Starting the day with one healthy action makes a second healthy action more likely, and a third more likely still. This is not metaphorical — behavioral science consistently demonstrates that initial actions lower the threshold for subsequent actions in the same direction. Drinking your morning water sets a different tone for breakfast than reaching immediately for coffee and scrolling your phone for forty minutes. Not because the water is pharmacologically capable of improving your breakfast choices, but because you have already made one choice that aligns with taking care of yourself, and maintaining that alignment feels natural and worth preserving.

Finally, rituals build self-trust. And for women who have cycled through years of starting and stopping wellness efforts, who have experienced the quiet erosion of confidence that comes from promising yourself you will change and then not sustaining the change, self-trust can be one of the most precious and depleted resources. Every morning that you complete your ritual, however simple, is a kept promise to yourself. And kept promises, accumulated day after day, rebuild the foundation of believing that you are capable of consistent self-care. That rebuilt self-trust then extends outward — making it easier to trust yourself around food, around exercise, around sleep, around all the other choices that shape your wellbeing.

The pink salt morning ritual is not important because of the minerals in the salt. It is important because of what it means, and what it builds, over time.

SODIUM, BLOATING, AND SMART USE

Given that this entire book is partly about reducing bloating, it would be incomplete — and not entirely honest — to discuss pink salt without addressing the complicated relationship between sodium and fluid retention.

Salt makes your body hold water. This is basic physiology, and it applies to pink Himalayan salt exactly as it applies to every other form of sodium chloride. When you consume sodium, your body works to maintain a specific ratio of sodium to water in the bloodstream, and if sodium intake increases, the body retains additional water to maintain that ratio. For most healthy people, in moderate amounts, this process is efficient and well-regulated. But it is real, and it matters in the context of bloating.

The quarter teaspoon of pink salt used in the morning ritual — which contains roughly 400 to 500 milligrams of sodium — is a modest amount. For most healthy women without specific medical considerations around sodium, this quantity in a glass of water is unlikely to cause problematic fluid retention, particularly because it is paired with hydrating water that actually supports the body's fluid balance overall. In fact, the mild electrolyte effect may, for many women, reduce the kind of water retention driven by dehydration and mineral imbalance.

However, context matters enormously. If you are also eating a diet that is high in sodium from processed foods, restaurant meals, packaged snacks, and condiments — which is very easy to do inadvertently in a modern food environment where sodium is used aggressively as a preservative and flavor enhancer — adding a pinch of pink salt to your morning water is a negligible addition to what may already be a high overall sodium picture. And high overall sodium intake does contribute to water retention, puffiness, and the kind of bloating that shows up as a swollen belly, tight rings, and a face that looks different in the mirror than it did a few days ago.

The most important principle here is not to obsess over the small amount of pink salt in your morning ritual but to develop broader awareness of where sodium is hiding in your daily eating. The worst culprits are typically packaged and processed foods — soups, sauces, deli meats, crackers, frozen meals, fast food — where sodium levels can be startlingly high without any obvious salty taste. Reading labels with sodium in mind, and gradually shifting toward a diet based more heavily on whole, unprocessed foods, will do far more for your bloating than any adjustments to your morning water.

Listening to your own body is also essential. Some women are more sensitive to sodium than others, and some days — particularly around hormonal fluctuations — your body may be more reactive to any additional sodium input. If you notice more puffiness or discomfort after your morning ritual on certain days, reduce the salt amount or skip it temporarily and observe. Your body is providing you with useful information. The goal is always to work with it, not override it.

WHO SHOULD BE CAUTIOUS

While the pink salt morning ritual is safe and appropriate for the vast majority of healthy women, there are circumstances in which a degree of caution or direct medical guidance is warranted, and this book would not be serving you honestly without addressing them.

If you have been diagnosed with high blood pressure, your physician or cardiologist may have recommended sodium restriction as part of managing your condition. While the amount of sodium in a single serving of morning salt water is relatively small, it is worth having a direct conversation with your healthcare provider about whether this addition to your routine is appropriate for your specific situation.

If you have kidney disease or impaired kidney function, your ability to regulate sodium and fluid balance may be compromised, and dietary sodium intake becomes more significant. Please consult your kidney specialist or primary care physician before adding any additional sodium to your daily routine.

If you are on medications that affect sodium or fluid balance — including certain blood pressure medications, diuretics, or corticosteroids — the interaction between those medications and additional sodium intake is something your prescribing physician should weigh in on.

If you have been given specific dietary sodium restrictions by any healthcare provider for any reason, those instructions take precedence over anything in this book, and you should discuss any modifications to your sodium intake with that provider before proceeding.

For the majority of readers — healthy women in their forties and fifties navigating hormonal transition without significant underlying conditions — the morning ritual as described is well within safe parameters. But responsible wellness guidance acknowledges that readers are individuals with individual health histories, and blanket recommendations cannot account for every circumstance. When in doubt, a conversation with your doctor or a registered dietitian will give you personalized guidance that this book cannot.

HOW TO CHOOSE A GOOD PINK SALT PRODUCT

Walk into almost any grocery store, health food shop, or browse online, and you will find pink Himalayan salt available at a remarkable range of prices — from a few dollars for a large bag to premium-packaged products that cost several times more for a fraction of the quantity.

The honest guidance here is refreshingly simple: for the purposes of the morning ritual and everyday use, an affordable, reputable pink Himalayan salt is entirely sufficient. You do not need the most expensive version. The mineral content does not vary dramatically between price points for genuine Himalayan salt, and the idea that a forty-dollar artisan salt provides meaningfully superior nutritional value compared to a five-dollar grocery store equivalent is, in most cases, creative marketing rather than substantiated fact.

What does matter is that you are buying actual pink Himalayan salt rather than a dyed or adulterated product. Genuine Himalayan salt should be labeled clearly as such, ideally with a country of origin that reflects Pakistan or the broader Himalayan region. The pink color should look natural and somewhat variable, with crystals ranging from pale to deeper rose rather than uniformly vivid or artificially bright. Reputable brands will often have third-party testing or certifications that support their quality claims.

Avoid products that attach extraordinary health claims to their salt — any packaging that promises hormonal balance, dramatic weight loss, or detoxification effects is prioritizing marketing over honesty, and that gap between promise and reality is exactly what this chapter has worked to close. The product itself may be perfectly fine salt; it is the claims that are the problem.

You can purchase fine-ground pink salt for dissolving in water, or coarser crystals that you grind yourself — either works well for the morning ritual. Fine-ground dissolves more readily, which makes it slightly more convenient for the morning routine when time is often limited.

Simplicity is the operating principle. Good quality, clean ingredient label, reasonable price, and the kind of straightforward product that does what it says without promising the impossible.

THE BIGGER PICTURE

Here is where everything comes into focus.

Pink salt, as you now understand, is a genuinely pleasant, mildly beneficial addition to a morning routine. It supports hydration in a practical, accessible way. It contributes trace minerals in small but real amounts. And perhaps most importantly, it serves as an anchor for a morning ritual that, practiced consistently, can be the beginning of a profound shift in how you care for yourself and how you feel in your body.

But the transformation you are looking for — the reduction in bloating that has you feeling heavy and uncomfortable, the sustained energy that seems to have gone missing, the sense of control around food that exhaustion and hormonal fluctuation have eroded, the lighter, more confident feeling in your own body — that transformation comes from the whole.

It comes from mornings that begin with intention rather than immediate stress. It comes from hydration that supports your body's fluid balance throughout the day. It comes from eating in a way that works with your hormones rather than against them — food that nourishes your muscle, stabilizes your blood sugar, and gives your gut what it needs to function smoothly. It comes from sleep that actually restores you. From movement that builds your metabolic foundation rather than depleting it. From practical, daily strategies for reducing the cortisol load that is quietly driving so much of what feels out of control.

The pink salt ritual is where this journey begins, because beginning matters. It matters to have a starting point that is simple, pleasurable, and immediately accessible — something you can do tomorrow morning that takes three minutes and costs almost nothing and begins to rebuild the daily self-care rhythm that everything else will build upon.

But it is a spark, not an engine. The engine is the full reset — the layered, practical, sustainable approach to supporting your body through this stage of life that the rest of this book will walk you through in detail.

In the next chapter, we are going to start building the morning ritual itself — not just the water and the salt, but the complete framework for a morning that sets up every hour that follows. Because the way you begin a day has an enormous influence on how that day unfolds, and the way you consistently begin your days has an enormous influence on your health, your energy, your body, and your sense of yourself.

You have the truth now. And the truth, it turns out, is more than enough to work with.

Let's build something real.

3

THE 5-MINUTE
MORNING RESET RITUAL

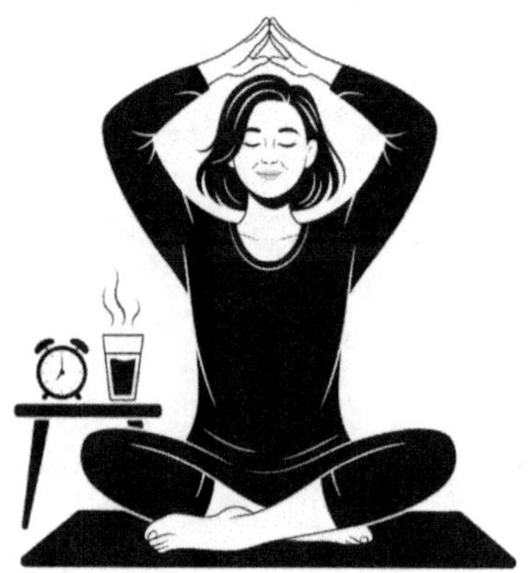

THINK ABOUT THE LAST TIME YOU HAD A GENUINELY GOOD MORNING.

Not a perfect morning, not the kind that only exists in magazines, where the light is golden and the coffee is already made and there is somehow an hour of quiet before the rest of the world wakes up. Just a good one. A morning where you woke up feeling reasonably rested, moved through the first hour with some sense of calm and purpose, made choices that felt nourishing rather than desperate, and arrived at mid-morning feeling like you were ahead of the day rather than already behind it.

How did the rest of that day tend to go?

Most women, when they think about this honestly, notice a pattern. The days that start well tend to continue well — not perfectly, but with a different quality of momentum. The food choices feel more considered. The stress feels more manageable. The energy holds a little longer. There is a thread of self-respect running through the hours that makes it easier to keep pulling in the same direction.

Now think about the opposite. The mornings that begin in a rush — alarm ignored too long, coffee grabbed while simultaneously checking messages, breakfast skipped or eaten standing over the sink, stress already elevated before you have left the house. Those days have a different quality too, and not a better one.

This is not coincidence, and it is not simply a matter of attitude. The way your morning unfolds has direct, measurable effects on your hormonal state, your blood sugar, your cortisol levels, and the neurological patterns that drive your choices for the rest of the day. How you begin matters — biologically, psychologically, and practically — far more than most wellness conversations acknowledge.

WHY MORNINGS MATTER MORE THAN YOU THINK

There is a window at the beginning of each day that is unlike any other. Before the demands arrive, before the notifications accumulate, before the needs of everyone and everything around you start pulling in competing directions — there is a brief period where you have the most access to yourself. Your attention is freshest. Your decision-making resources are least depleted. The neurological slate has been, to some degree, reset by sleep.

What you do in that window sets the physiological and psychological tone for everything that follows.

From a hormonal perspective, the morning is when cortisol naturally peaks. This is by design — the cortisol awakening response, as researchers call it, is your body's built-in alarm system, producing a surge of cortisol in the first thirty to forty-five minutes after waking to mobilize energy, sharpen alertness, and prepare you for the demands of the day. In a healthy, well-regulated system, this morning cortisol peak is beneficial. It creates drive and focus.

The problem arises when you add significant additional stressors to an already activated stress system. Checking your phone immediately upon waking floods your brain with information, demands, and emotional triggers before you have had a chance to regulate. Rushing without eating or eating something that spikes and crashes blood sugar sends your metabolic system into a reactive state. Skipping hydration after a night of fasting means your body is operating in a mildly dehydrated state that impairs cognitive function and intensifies the physiological stress response.

The result, for many women, is a morning cortisol peak that becomes a cortisol spike — an elevated stress response that does not settle back down cleanly but instead carries a residue of activation into the rest of the day. And elevated cortisol through the morning and afternoon, as we discussed in the previous chapter, promotes abdominal fat storage, intensifies cravings for sugar and salt, disrupts digestion, and erodes the calm clarity that makes good choices feel easy rather than effortful.

For women in perimenopause and menopause, this dynamic is amplified. Declining progesterone means less of the naturally calming, GABA-activating hormonal influence that once took the edge off a stressful morning. Declining estrogen means less natural buffering of the cortisol stress response. The nervous system is, in a very real sense, running with less of its original shock absorption — which means the quality of how you begin your day has an even greater impact than it did in your thirties.

A chaotic morning does not just feel bad. For a body navigating hormonal transition, it creates a biochemical environment that works directly against the goals of feeling lighter, more energized, less bloated, and more in control. And conversely, a morning that begins with even a few minutes of calm intention creates a meaningfully different starting point — one where cortisol rises and settles naturally, where hydration is established early, where your nervous system receives a signal of safety and ease rather than urgency and threat.

You do not need an extra hour to create this. You need five minutes. And those five minutes, repeated consistently, will change more than you might currently believe is possible from something so small.

THE POWER OF A 5-MINUTE RITUAL

There is a particular kind of discouragement that comes from wellness approaches that are simply too much for real life.

You have probably felt it. The meal plan that requires four hours of Sunday preparation. The workout program that demands six days a week. The morning routine you read about that involves oil pulling, journaling, meditation, cold showers, yoga, and a smoothie made from seventeen ingredients. These approaches are not wrong, exactly — many of the individual components are genuinely beneficial. But for a woman who is already managing a full and demanding life, the gap between the recommended ideal and what is actually executable on a Tuesday morning is often so wide that the whole thing collapses under its own weight before it has a chance to take root.

Small habits are different. They are different not because they are less powerful, but because they are actually sustainable — and sustainability, as we have discussed, is the foundation of all meaningful progress.

Behavioral researchers who study habit formation have found consistently that the most reliable predictor of whether a habit will be maintained is not its perceived importance or even the motivation of the person practicing it. It is friction — the degree of effort, complexity, and disruption required to perform the behavior. Habits that require minimal friction get done. Habits that require navigating multiple barriers, acquiring special equipment, or carving out significant time from an already packed schedule get abandoned, regardless of how much you wanted them to work.

A five-minute morning ritual has almost no friction. The ingredients are simple and inexpensive. The preparation takes moments. The practice itself requires no special skill, no equipment, no perfect conditions. You can do it in a small kitchen while children are waking up. You can do it in a hotel room while traveling. You can do it on the mornings when you are tired, when you are stressed, when you are running late — because it takes five minutes, and almost all mornings have five minutes somewhere in them.

And here is the transformative part: because you can do it on the hard days as well as the easy ones, you will do it. And doing it consistently, across weeks and months, creates something that no elaborate protocol abandoned after ten days ever can: a track record. Evidence, accumulated in your own experience, that you are someone who follows through. That you keep promises to yourself. That you have a practice — however modest — that you maintain.

That track record is worth more than it sounds. For many women who have cycled through ambitious starts and frustrated stops, the quiet rebuilding of self-trust that comes from a kept daily promise is genuinely healing. It changes the internal narrative from "I always start strong and fail" to "I do this every day." And that changed narrative makes every subsequent healthy choice feel more like an extension of who you are rather than an effortful departure from your default.

Five minutes. Every morning. That is where this begins.

THE CORE PINK SALT MORNING RITUAL

The ritual itself is beautifully simple, and that simplicity is intentional. Here is exactly how to do it.

Begin with water — roughly eight to twelve ounces, which is a standard glass or mug. The temperature matters less than you might have been led to believe by various wellness sources, but warm or room-temperature water tends to be gentler on the digestive system first thing in the morning than cold water straight from the refrigerator, particularly for women who experience digestive sensitivity. Cold water can cause a mild constriction of the digestive tract, while warm water tends to be soothing and may support gentle morning gut motility. Use whichever feels comfortable and appealing to you.

Add a small pinch of pink Himalayan salt — approximately one quarter teaspoon or slightly less. You do not need to measure precisely. A modest, rounded pinch from your fingers is close enough, and you will develop a feel for the right amount after a few mornings. The salt should dissolve easily in warm water with a gentle stir.

If you enjoy lemon — and many women find it both pleasant and settling for their digestion — add a squeeze of fresh lemon juice from a quarter to half a lemon. Lemon adds a brightness to the flavor that many people find more appealing than plain salted water, and the citric acid has a mildly alkalizing effect after digestion and may support the production of digestive enzymes. It is not essential, but it is a genuinely nice addition if it appeals to you.

Stir gently. That is the preparation — two ingredients, thirty seconds.

Now, and this is the part that distinguishes the ritual from simply drinking a glass of water: drink it with intention. Not while scrolling your phone. Not while simultaneously making lunches or answering messages. Before any of that. Take your glass somewhere you can be still for a few minutes — your kitchen table, a chair by a window, your garden or porch if the weather allows — and drink slowly, in the quiet of a morning that has not yet fully started.

This deliberate, unhurried quality is not precious or self-indulgent. It is physiologically relevant. Drinking in a calm state allows your body to actually absorb and use the hydration effectively. Your digestive system is more receptive to fluids when your parasympathetic nervous system — your rest and digest state — is active, rather than when you are rushing in a stress response. Those few quiet minutes of drinking your morning ritual water are not incidental to the practice. They are part of it.

Try to do this before your first coffee or tea, and before eating breakfast. Hydrating before caffeine is particularly valuable, because caffeine has a mild diuretic effect and consuming it before your body has been rehydrated from the night means you are further depleting hydration before establishing it. Even a ten-minute gap between your ritual water and your first coffee is beneficial.

The whole process — preparing, drinking, the quiet minutes — takes five minutes. Often slightly less. It is the easiest significant thing you will do for your health today.

OPTIONAL RITUAL VARIATIONS

The core ritual is the foundation, and you are encouraged to begin with it exactly as described and give it time to become automatic before adding any complexity. But real life is varied, taste preferences differ, and some days call for adjustments. Here are several variations to know about, offered as options rather than upgrades.

The lemon and ginger version adds a small amount of fresh grated ginger — about a quarter teaspoon — to the core recipe. Ginger is one of the most well-researched natural digestive supporters available, with genuine evidence for reducing nausea, supporting gut motility, and reducing inflammation in the digestive tract. If bloating and digestive discomfort are particularly prominent for you, especially in the morning, this variation is worth trying. The flavor is warming and slightly spicy, which many women find especially welcome on cooler mornings.

The apple cider vinegar version adds a teaspoon of raw, unfiltered apple cider vinegar — the kind with the cloudy sediment, often labeled "with the mother" — to the core recipe. Apple cider vinegar has attracted considerable wellness attention, and while the more dramatic claims about its effects are overstated, there is reasonable evidence that the acetic acid in apple cider vinegar may support modest improvements in blood sugar regulation and digestive enzyme activity. If you try this variation, start with a small amount — half a teaspoon — as the acidity can be strong for some people, and always dilute it well in water. Never drink it undiluted.

The travel version is for the mornings when you are away from home and do not have your usual supplies. A small travel container of pink salt takes up almost no space in a bag and can be dissolved in a glass of bottled or tap water in any hotel room, at any airport, on any early morning when your routine is disrupted. Having a plan for how to maintain your ritual while traveling removes one of the most common reasons habits collapse — the interruption of the familiar environment.

The salt-free hydration version is for any morning when you prefer not to add salt — whether because of a lower-sodium day, a medical consideration, a personal preference, or simply a morning when plain warm lemon water feels more appealing. Drinking a large glass of warm water first thing in the morning, even without any additions, is deeply valuable. The ritual is about the intention and the hydration as much as it is about any specific ingredient. Do not let the absence of one component be a reason to skip the practice entirely.

The ultra-busy two-minute version exists for the mornings that are genuinely impossible — the alarm-overslept, school-run-in-ten-minutes, absolute-chaos mornings that every woman's life contains. Keep a small glass on your bathroom counter. Fill it with water, add a pinch of salt from a container you keep right there beside it, drink it before you do anything else. Sixty seconds. It is enough. The ritual is maintained, the streak continues, and you have given your body something even in the hardest morning. That matters.

ADD A BODY RESET IN MOTION

The morning water ritual is the centerpiece of this daily reset, but if you can add even one small movement practice immediately afterward — before the day fully begins and before the demands take over — you will compound the benefits considerably.

Movement in the morning does several things that are particularly valuable for women over forty. It activates your muscles before a day of sitting, which supports your metabolic rate and blood sugar management throughout the day. It reduces morning cortisol more effectively than staying still, helping your stress hormonal curve settle into a healthy pattern. It supports lymphatic flow and circulation, which directly reduces the overnight puffiness and water retention that can feel demoralizing first thing in the morning. And it establishes a second kept promise to yourself before eight in the morning, which builds the momentum that makes the rest of the day feel more possible.

The movement does not need to be vigorous, and for the purposes of this morning ritual, it is better if it is not. This is not the time for your most intense workout — that can happen later in the day if it suits your schedule and your body. This is a gentle activation, a way of waking up the body and inviting circulation and ease rather than demanding performance.

A ten-minute walk outside is perhaps the most valuable option available to most women. Walking in natural daylight first thing in the morning does something that nothing else quite replicates: it entrains your circadian rhythm by exposing your eyes to natural light during the critical window that sets your internal clock for the day. This has downstream effects on your evening melatonin production, your sleep quality, and the natural cortisol curve that governs your energy throughout the day. Even on cloudy days, the light intensity outside is significantly greater than indoor lighting and sufficient to activate these biological processes.

If a walk is not possible, five minutes of gentle movement in your living space is genuinely worthwhile. Simple hip circles, shoulder rolls, a few slow squats, a gentle forward fold, cat-cow stretches on the floor — movements that take your joints through their range of motion and wake up the muscles without demanding much from a system that is still transitioning from sleep. Many women find that this kind of gentle morning movement reduces the stiffness and heaviness that can make mornings feel laborious, creating a physical lightness that carries into the rest of the day.

Deep breathing — even five slow, deliberate cycles of breath while standing with your feet on the ground, ideally outside — activates the parasympathetic nervous system in measurable ways, lowering cortisol, reducing heart rate, and establishing a baseline of calm that makes everything else easier. It takes about ninety seconds, it requires no equipment, and the physiological effects are real.

Choose whatever form of movement feels accessible and appealing to you, commit to doing it immediately after your ritual water for twenty-one days, and observe what changes. The combination of hydration and gentle movement in the first twenty minutes of your morning is among the most powerful and underutilized tools available to women navigating midlife hormonal change.

THE MINDSET MINUTE

There is one more component of the morning reset that belongs here, even though it requires nothing physical and produces no measurable biochemical change: the mindset minute.

Before the ritual is complete, take sixty seconds — just sixty — for a simple mental practice that shifts your internal orientation from reactive to intentional. This is not a demand for elaborate journaling or a complicated visualization exercise. It is one small moment of deliberate thought before the day takes over completely.

It might look like this: while you are finishing your glass of water, or in the moments immediately after, you bring one thought to the surface. Not a goal, not a to-do list, not a worry you are already carrying from yesterday. One simple thing you are genuinely glad about. One thing about this specific morning, or your life, or your body, or the day ahead that carries even a small charge of gratitude or positive anticipation.

This is not toxic positivity. It is not pretending that everything is fine when it is not, or forcing cheerfulness over genuine difficulty. It is simply the deliberate activation of a neural pathway — because gratitude and positive anticipation, however briefly held, genuinely shift the neurological and hormonal context of the moment that follows. Even a modest gratitude practice, practiced consistently, has been shown in behavioral and neurological research to reduce baseline cortisol, improve mood, and increase the likelihood of sustained positive behavior.

You can also use this minute to set a single intention for the day. Not a list of achievements. One orientation. Something like: today I will eat in a way that makes me feel good. Today I will move gently and with kindness toward my body. Today I will notice when I am stressed and take a breath before I reach for food. The specifics are less important than the act of arriving at the day with some conscious direction rather than simply being swept forward by whatever comes.

Many women find it helpful to add a single sentence of spoken or mental self-compassion to this minute — a brief acknowledgment that yesterday is over, that whatever happened or did not happen, this morning is a fresh beginning, and that they are doing their best in a genuinely complex season of life. The self-blame and guilt that many women carry around their health and their bodies is one of the most reliable saboteurs of progress, because guilt activates the same stress pathways that drive the very behaviors you are trying to change. Even thirty seconds of consciously releasing yesterday's imperfect choices and choosing a different orientation today is physiologically meaningful, not just emotionally.

Sixty seconds. One grateful thought, one intention, one moment of self-compassion. The day you step into after that minute is genuinely different from the one you would have stepped into without it.

HOW TO MAKE THE RITUAL AUTOMATIC

The gap between a habit you intend to start and a habit that actually becomes automatic is bridged by design, not willpower. If the ritual requires you to remember it, find the ingredients, make a decision, and overcome inertia every single morning, it will eventually fail — not because you lack commitment, but because willpower is finite and mornings are unpredictable. The solution is to engineer your environment so that the ritual is the path of least resistance.

The most effective single strategy is to prepare your supplies the night before. Keep your pink salt in a small container right next to the kettle or wherever you make your morning water. Put your glass on the counter before you go to bed. If you use lemon, cut it the night before and keep it ready in the refrigerator. When you wake up, everything you need is already assembled and waiting. The ritual requires no searching, no decision-making, no friction.

Habit stacking — the practice of linking a new habit to an existing one — is one of the most reliable techniques from behavioral science for building new behaviors. Identify something you already do every single morning without exception: perhaps you turn on the kettle, or you go to the bathroom, or you feed a pet. Decide that the pink salt water ritual happens immediately after that existing action, every time, without deliberation. Over time, the existing habit triggers the new one automatically, removing the need for conscious intention entirely.

Physical visibility is a surprisingly powerful cue. When your pink salt container is sitting on your counter in plain sight, it serves as a passive reminder that requires no cognitive effort. When it is tucked in a cupboard, behind other things, requiring you to remember and retrieve it, it creates friction. Keep everything you need for this ritual where you can see it. The environment that makes healthy behavior easy is one of the most impactful changes you can make.

Consider keeping a simple record of your practice for the first twenty-one days — not an elaborate tracker, just a small mark in a notebook or on a calendar for each morning completed. The visual accumulation of consecutive marks creates what behavioral researchers call a "don't break the chain" effect, where the desire to maintain a growing streak becomes itself a motivating force. Many women find that on the mornings when they feel least like making the effort, glancing at a row of consecutive marks is enough to carry them through.

Make the ritual enjoyable enough that you look forward to it. Use a glass or mug you genuinely like. Create a few minutes of quiet that are genuinely pleasant — perhaps near a window, with some soft light, before anyone else is awake. The more your brain associates the ritual with positive sensory and emotional experience, the more reliably it will pull you toward the behavior rather than requiring you to push.

WHAT IF YOU MISS A DAY?

You will miss a day. At some point — a morning so hectic that the ritual simply does not happen, a night of disrupted sleep that has you running late and barely functional, a period of travel or illness or family crisis — you will wake up and the ritual will not have been completed by the time the morning is over.

This is not a problem. It is an inevitability, and planning for it in advance is part of building a practice that actually lasts.

The single most important rule for navigating a missed day is simple: never miss twice in a row. One missed day is a minor interruption in an ongoing practice. Two missed days in a row is the beginning of a gap that can quietly grow into a week, and then a month, before you realize the habit has dissolved. The moment you recognize that yesterday was missed is the moment to commit, firmly and without drama, to today.

Not a restart. Not a new beginning with renewed determination and a fresh page. Just a return — quiet, unremarkable, immediate. You missed yesterday. Today you drink your water. That is all.

The perfectionism that makes women declare an entire effort failed over a single skipped day is one of the most destructive patterns in wellness culture, and it is so deeply ingrained that most women do not even notice they are doing it. The internal logic goes something like this: the streak is broken, therefore the effort is compromised, therefore there is less reason to continue, therefore I might as well start fresh on Monday. And Monday becomes next week, and next week becomes next month, and the precious momentum of consistent practice is lost — not because of the missed day, but because of the story told about it.

A single missed day does not undo a week of practice. Two missed days in a row do not undo a month. Your body does not forget the hydration it has received, the habits it has begun forming, the morning cortisol patterns that have started shifting. Habits exist in a continuum, not an on-off switch, and a brief interruption followed by an immediate return leaves far less residue than the catastrophizing that turns one imperfect morning into an abandoned practice.

Treat yourself with the same kindness you would offer a friend. If your friend told you she had missed her morning ritual yesterday, you would not tell her she had failed and should start over. You would tell her it does not matter and to just do it today. Offer yourself the same grace. It is not weakness. It is the practical wisdom that makes long-term consistency actually achievable.

YOUR FIRST 21 DAYS

There is something meaningful about the number twenty-one in the context of habit formation — not because habits are automatically fixed and permanent at day twenty-two, which is an oversimplification of more complex neuroscience, but because three weeks of consistent practice is generally enough to move from deliberate effort to something closer to automatic. It is enough time to notice real changes. It is enough time to begin experiencing the ritual as part of your identity rather than a new thing you are trying.

Here is an honest picture of what those twenty-one days tend to look like.

The first week often has the quality of a beginning — the combination of novelty and genuine effort that makes a new habit feel both promising and slightly effortful. You may notice some immediate effects: many women report feeling more awake within a day or two of establishing proper morning hydration, simply because they have been beginning their days in a state of mild dehydration for years and the contrast is immediately noticeable. Digestion may feel slightly more mobile, and the sluggish heaviness that often characterizes mornings may begin to lift a little. Energy in the first few hours of the day may improve.

You may also notice, during the first week, that some mornings you feel distinctly unimpressive. That the ritual feels mechanical and uninspiring, that you do not feel particularly different, that a voice in your head wonders whether this is really worth the bother. This is entirely normal. Week one is about establishing the pattern, not experiencing a transformation. Give it more time.

By the second week, the ritual typically begins requiring less conscious effort. You find yourself moving toward the kettle and the salt container without quite deciding to — the behavioral groove is forming. You may begin to notice your mornings feeling slightly more anchored, the transition from waking to functioning slightly smoother. If you have added the morning movement component, your body may begin to feel a mild but real difference in morning stiffness and overall physical ease.

Pay attention during the second week to how your mornings compare to days when you have not yet completed the ritual. Many women notice, with growing clarity, that the days beginning with the ritual simply feel different — not dramatically, but in the kind of small, consistent way that compounds into meaningful wellbeing over time.

The third week tends to be where something shifts more noticeably. Not necessarily in a dramatic, measurable way — though some women do notice visible changes in morning bloating, energy consistency, and the quality of their food choices throughout the day — but in a quieter, more fundamental way. The ritual has become something you do, not something you are trying to do. And that distinction carries a weight that is hard to describe but immediately recognizable: it is the feeling of a practice that has become genuinely yours.

Watch for small wins and take them seriously, because they are the real measure of progress in these early weeks. The morning that begins with the ritual and leads naturally to a nourishing breakfast. The afternoon when the usual energy crash does not arrive with its usual intensity. The evening when you notice you have drunk more water than usual without any particular effort. The moment when you realize you have completed twenty-one consecutive mornings and something in you has quietly, persistently changed.

These are not small things. They are the building blocks of the transformation this book is designed to help you create — one gentle, consistent, accumulated morning at a time.

The ritual is established. Now it is time to nourish the body that surrounds it. In the next chapter, we will move into the food strategies that work with your hormones rather than against them — the practical, sustainable approach to eating that supports everything the morning ritual has begun to build.

You have started. Keep going.

4

BEAT BELLY BLOAT AND
FEEL LIGHTER FAST

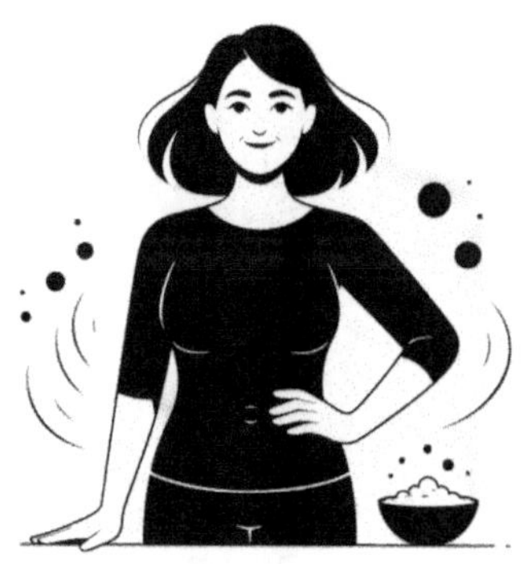

THERE IS A PARTICULAR KIND OF FRUSTRATION THAT ARRIVES IN THE EVENING.

You woke up feeling reasonably okay — maybe even a little lighter than usual, encouraged by how your waistband felt when you got dressed. You made reasonable choices through the day. You drank your water. You tried. And then, somewhere between lunch and dinner, the familiar tightness crept back in. By early evening, your stomach feels distended and uncomfortable, your clothes feel confining in a way they did not this morning, and the mirror shows something that looks and feels very different from the version of you that started the day.

If you have experienced this cycle — the morning-to-evening transformation that can make you feel like your body is working against you in real time — you are in very good company. It is one of the most commonly reported physical frustrations among women over forty, and it is one of the most emotionally exhausting, precisely because it is so visible and so persistent and because it so often gets mistaken for something it is not.

That misidentification is where a great deal of unnecessary suffering begins. Because the bloating and puffiness that so many women experience — that swollen, heavy, tight feeling that can add what looks like several inches to your midsection over the course of a day — is not the same thing as fat gain. It does not mean you are failing. It does not mean the weight is coming back, or that your efforts are pointless, or that your body is irreparably changed. It means something specific is happening in your physiology that can be understood, addressed, and significantly improved.

This chapter is going to show you exactly how.

WHY BLOATING FEELS SO DEFEATING

Before we get into the mechanics of what bloating actually is and what drives it, it is worth spending a moment with the emotional reality of living with it. Because the physical discomfort is real, but the psychological weight of chronic bloating is something that does not always get enough acknowledgment.

Clothes that fit in the morning and do not fit by afternoon create a particular kind of anxiety that follows you through the day. You begin choosing what to wear based not on what you like but on what has enough give to accommodate the swelling you know is coming. You turn down invitations to events where you will be photographed, or where you know you will be standing and talking and feeling self-conscious about your middle. You develop a complicated relationship with your wardrobe — a drawer full of clothes you love but rarely wear because they are unforgiving on the days you feel puffiest, which increasingly feels like most days.

There is also the scale confusion. You weigh yourself in the morning and the number is one thing; you weigh yourself in the evening and it can be two, three, or even four pounds higher. You know intellectually that you have not gained three pounds of fat in a single day, and yet the visual and physical evidence of your expanding midsection makes that rational knowledge hard to hold onto. The number becomes loaded with emotion, and the emotion makes it almost impossible to interpret the information clearly.

Many women in their forties and fifties tell themselves that the bloating they experience is simply how their body looks now — that it is fat, that it is permanent, that the battle is already lost. This belief leads to a particular kind of resignation that is both understandable and genuinely unnecessary. Because bloating, in most cases, is not permanent. It is dynamic. It changes from day to day, from morning to evening, in response to identifiable factors that you have more influence over than you may currently believe.

Understanding what is actually happening is the first and most powerful step toward changing it.

FAT VERSUS BLOAT: UNDERSTANDING THE DIFFERENCE

The distinction between actual body fat and bloating sounds simple in theory but can feel almost impossible to hold onto in practice, especially when you are living in a body that looks and feels different from day to day in ways that seem random and uncontrollable.

Body fat is tissue — specifically, adipose tissue, which is composed of fat cells that store energy in the form of lipids. It accumulates gradually, over weeks and months, in response to a sustained excess of energy consumed relative to energy expended, along with hormonal signals that influence where and how readily fat is stored. It does not appear overnight, and it does not disappear overnight. Changes in actual body fat are slow, consistent, and relatively stable from day to day.

Bloating is something entirely different. It is a temporary increase in the volume or perceived firmness of the abdomen caused by one of several distinct mechanisms: gas accumulation in the digestive tract, water retention in the tissues, slowed gut motility that causes contents to sit longer than usual, or a combination of all three. None of these mechanisms involve the addition of fat tissue, and none of them produce changes that are permanent or even particularly slow to reverse when their underlying causes are addressed.

When you wake up looking leaner and by evening feel as though your stomach has doubled in size, what you are experiencing is almost certainly not fat gain — it is the accumulation of gas, fluid, and digestive contents over the course of the day. This is a normal biological process, and some degree of it happens in every body. The issue for many women over forty is that the degree has increased, the causes have become more numerous, and the body's ability to resolve the bloating overnight has become less efficient.

Water retention is a closely related phenomenon that deserves its own moment of attention. Fluid is held in the spaces between cells — the interstitial tissue — in amounts that vary significantly based on hormonal levels, sodium intake, hydration status, inflammatory load, and a range of other factors. When fluid retention is elevated, it shows up as puffiness in the face and hands and feet, a feeling of heaviness throughout the body, and a tighter, more swollen appearance in the abdomen. The number on the scale goes up — sometimes dramatically — and yet none of it is fat. It is water, responding to the conditions your body is currently operating under.

This matters enormously for how you interpret your progress. The scale measures everything — fat, muscle, water, the contents of your digestive tract, the food you have not yet digested. Treating its daily fluctuations as meaningful data about fat gain or loss will consistently mislead you. A woman who has been eating well, hydrating properly, and moving consistently may step on the scale on a day of high water retention and see a number that appears to have undone a week of effort — and none of it reflects her actual progress. Learning to separate the signal from the noise, and to measure your wellbeing by how you feel and how your clothes fit over time rather than by a daily number, is one of the most liberating shifts you can make on this journey.

WHY BLOATING OFTEN INCREASES AFTER 40

If you feel like your bloating has become noticeably worse since your late thirties or early forties, you are not imagining the change. There are real, specific reasons why bloating tends to increase during perimenopause and menopause, and understanding them transforms the experience from something mysterious and demoralizing into something logical and workable.

Hormonal fluctuation is the starting point. Estrogen and progesterone both influence gut function directly. Estrogen receptors exist throughout the gastrointestinal tract, and as estrogen levels fluctuate and eventually decline, gut motility — the coordinated muscular contractions that move food through the digestive system — can slow significantly. Food that moves through the intestines more slowly has more time to ferment, producing more gas and more of the tightness and distension that characterizes bloating. This is not a digestive dysfunction, strictly speaking. It is a normal adaptation to a changed hormonal environment. But it does mean that your gut is genuinely working differently than it was before.

Progesterone's decline has its own contribution. Progesterone relaxes smooth muscle tissue, including the smooth muscle of the intestinal walls. When progesterone falls, this relaxation effect is reduced, which can create more variability in how the digestive tract moves — sometimes too slow, sometimes with urgency, and often with more gas and discomfort than was previously typical.

Cortisol, which we have discussed at length in earlier chapters, has a direct and significant impact on gut function. The gut and the brain are in constant bidirectional communication through what researchers call the gut-brain axis — a network of nerves, hormones, and signaling molecules that links the emotional and cognitive centers of the brain to the intestinal environment. When cortisol is elevated, digestion is suppressed, gut motility changes, the balance of bacteria in the gut microbiome shifts, and the gut lining can become more permeable — all of which contribute to increased bloating, gas, and digestive discomfort.

Poor sleep, which becomes increasingly common during perimenopause, adds another layer. Sleep is when the gut performs a significant amount of its repair and regulatory work, and when sleep quality is consistently disrupted, the gut microbiome shifts toward compositions associated with more gas production, more inflammation, and less efficient digestion.

The gut microbiome itself — the vast community of bacteria that inhabits your intestinal tract and performs an enormous range of functions related to digestion, immunity, inflammation, and even mood — is sensitive to the hormonal changes of menopause in ways that are only beginning to be well understood. Research suggests that the composition of the gut microbiome changes meaningfully during this transition, often in directions that reduce the bacterial diversity that is associated with healthy digestion and comfortable gut function.

Food sensitivities that may not have been significant in your thirties can become more pronounced in your forties, as the combination of changed gut permeability, altered microbiome composition, and reduced digestive enzyme production creates a landscape where foods that were once well-tolerated begin producing symptoms. Dairy, wheat, and certain high-fermentable carbohydrates are common examples, though the specific sensitivities vary considerably between individuals.

Less daily movement — which tends to accompany the life stage of many women in their forties and fifties, with busier schedules, more desk-based work, and less spontaneous physical activity than earlier decades — directly affects gut motility. Physical movement stimulates the mechanical movement of the digestive tract, and when overall activity levels decline, digestion slows and gas accumulates more readily.

Understanding this landscape is not meant to make the situation feel overwhelming. Quite the opposite. Each of these factors is something you have some degree of influence over — and the strategies in this chapter are designed to address them in practical, manageable ways.

COMMON FOOD AND LIFESTYLE TRIGGERS

While the hormonal and physiological context of midlife creates a background of increased bloating susceptibility, specific daily triggers often determine how pronounced the bloating is on any given day. Identifying your personal triggers is one of the most practical and immediately impactful things you can do to reduce bloating, and it begins with awareness rather than elimination.

Highly processed and packaged foods are among the most consistent bloating triggers across the population. They are typically high in sodium, which drives water retention. They often contain emulsifiers, stabilizers, and artificial sweeteners — particularly sugar alcohols like sorbitol and maltitol — that the gut bacteria ferment enthusiastically, producing significant gas. And they are frequently low in fiber and whole food compounds that support healthy gut motility. The combination creates conditions that are almost optimized for bloating, and many women find that even modest reductions in processed food intake produce noticeable improvements in digestive comfort within a few days.

Eating speed is profoundly underestimated as a bloating factor. When you eat quickly, you swallow a significant amount of air alongside your food — air that then accumulates in the digestive tract and contributes directly to gas and distension. Fast eating also means less thorough chewing, which means larger food particles arriving in the stomach where they require more digestive work, longer transit times, and more opportunity for fermentation. Slowing down and chewing thoroughly does not require extra time at the table — it simply requires a different quality of attention during the time you are already spending eating.

Carbonated drinks introduce gas directly into the digestive tract. For many women, regular consumption of sparkling water, diet sodas, or carbonated beverages is a significant but easily overlooked contributor to bloating. This does not mean sparkling water is forbidden territory, but if you are experiencing significant bloating and consuming carbonated beverages regularly, reducing them temporarily and observing the effect is a straightforward experiment.

Eating large meals, particularly in the evenings when digestion naturally slows, overwhelms the digestive system's capacity to process food efficiently. The result is food sitting in the digestive tract for extended periods, fermenting, producing gas, and creating the overnight bloating that makes mornings feel heavy and swollen. Redistributing your food intake toward earlier in the day and keeping evening meals lighter is one of the most consistently effective strategies for waking up feeling flatter and more comfortable.

Alcohol, in addition to its other effects on hormonal health, irritates the gut lining directly and disrupts the gut microbiome in ways that can produce significant bloating and digestive discomfort. Many women over forty notice that their digestive response to alcohol has become more pronounced than it was in earlier years — a reflection of both the changed gut environment and reduced enzyme production.

Inadequate water intake throughout the day contributes to constipation, which slows the movement of gas and waste through the digestive system and directly worsens bloating. Ironically, many women who are bloated instinctively reduce their water intake, believing that less fluid will mean less swelling — but the opposite is true. Proper hydration supports gut motility and actually reduces the water retention driven by dehydration.

Stress eating — consuming food quickly and in large amounts in response to emotional activation rather than genuine hunger — combines many of the worst bloating triggers simultaneously: fast eating with air swallowing, large volume, often processed comfort foods, and a gut that is already in a state of compromised function due to elevated cortisol. Developing awareness of stress eating patterns, without judgment, is the first step toward interrupting the cycle.

HIDDEN SODIUM AND PUFFINESS

It is worth returning briefly to sodium here, because the relationship between salt and puffiness is real and it matters — but it is easily misunderstood in ways that create unnecessary anxiety around the wrong things.

The pink salt morning ritual contains a modest and intentional amount of sodium, delivered in a hydrating context that most healthy women tolerate well. That is not the sodium to worry about. The sodium that drives the kind of persistent, day-long puffiness that many women experience comes from a very different source: the cumulative, largely invisible sodium in packaged and processed foods that has become the background noise of a modern diet.

A single serving of canned soup can contain over a thousand milligrams of sodium. A portion of restaurant food can easily contain two thousand milligrams or more. Salad dressings, condiments, bread, crackers, frozen meals, deli meats — even foods that do not taste particularly salty can carry significant sodium loads. And because the daily recommended sodium intake for most adults is around two thousand three hundred milligrams, it is remarkably easy to exceed that amount by lunchtime without having added a single pinch of salt to anything.

The practical guidance here is not to become obsessive about reading labels or calculating exact sodium intake — that level of vigilance is neither enjoyable nor sustainable. It is simply to develop a general awareness of where the largest sodium loads in your current diet are coming from, and to make gradual shifts toward meals built more heavily around whole, unprocessed foods, where the sodium content is naturally lower and more within your control.

Cooking from whole ingredients even a few times per week, replacing highly processed convenience foods with simpler alternatives, and paying occasional attention to sodium on nutrition labels when choosing packaged products are all practical ways to reduce your background sodium load without making food feel like a minefield. The goal is informed awareness, not anxiety. Your body responds to patterns over time, not to individual choices in isolation.

GUT-FRIENDLY DAILY HABITS

Beyond the removal or reduction of triggers, there are specific daily habits that actively support digestive health, reduce gas and fermentation in the gut, and create the internal conditions for feeling lighter and more comfortable. None of these habits are extreme or time-consuming. They are the kind of small, consistent practices that compound into significant change when maintained over weeks and months.

Chewing food thoroughly is the most undervalued digestive habit available to you, and it costs nothing except a small adjustment in attention. Digestion begins in the mouth, where enzymes in saliva begin breaking down carbohydrates and where mechanical chewing reduces food to particles small enough for efficient stomach processing. When food arrives in the stomach insufficiently chewed, the downstream fermentation and gas production increase considerably. Aiming to chew each bite until it is genuinely smooth before swallowing — more chewing than feels natural if you are accustomed to eating quickly — produces measurable improvements in digestive comfort for many women.

Eating regular meals at consistent times supports the gut's circadian biology. Your digestive system has its own internal clock, and it performs best when it receives food at predictable intervals rather than in irregular, sporadic patterns. Skipping meals and then eating very large amounts later disrupts this rhythm and creates exactly the kind of large, fermentable food load that produces significant bloating. Three balanced meals, or two meals and one smaller snack, eaten at roughly consistent times each day, is a pattern that tends to support stable digestion for most women.

Walking after meals is one of the most evidence-supported simple strategies for reducing post-meal bloating. Even a ten-to-fifteen-minute gentle walk stimulates the mechanical movement of the digestive tract, helps gas move through and dissipate, reduces post-meal blood sugar spikes, and supports the overall motility that keeps the system moving efficiently. It requires no equipment, no special clothing, and produces results that many women notice within the first few days of making it a habit.

Hydration throughout the day — not just at breakfast, but as a consistent background practice — keeps the digestive contents moving, reduces constipation, and prevents the fluid retention that comes from chronic mild dehydration. Carrying water with you, placing glasses of water in visible locations, and developing the habit of drinking water before coffee, before meals, and during the afternoon hours between meals are all practical ways to build better hydration without it requiring significant effort.

Fiber balance is worth particular attention. Fiber is genuinely important for gut health, healthy cholesterol levels, blood sugar stability, and digestive regularity — but both too little and too much fiber, or a sudden dramatic increase in fiber intake, can cause or worsen bloating. The goal is a consistent, moderate intake of fiber from a variety of sources — vegetables, legumes, whole grains, fruits — rather than either the very low fiber of a highly processed diet or the abrupt addition of large amounts of fiber-rich foods in an attempt to improve digestion quickly.

Reducing chronic stress, which we have discussed extensively in earlier chapters, is also directly a gut health intervention. The connection between psychological stress and digestive symptoms is not metaphorical — it is physiological, mediated by the gut-brain axis. Practices that reduce the chronic activation of your stress response — the morning mindset minute, gentle movement, adequate sleep, moments of deliberate rest during the day

— are simultaneously practices that support gut function and reduce bloating.

EVENING HABITS FOR A FLATTER MORNING

The quality of how you sleep and what you do in the hours before bed has an enormous influence on how you feel when you wake up — and specifically on whether you wake up with the relative flatness that makes the morning feel like a fresh start, or the overnight bloating and puffiness that casts a shadow before the day has even begun.

Keeping your evening meal lighter than your lunch is one of the most consistently effective strategies for reducing morning bloating. The body's digestive capacity naturally decreases as the day progresses, and a large, heavy dinner eaten late in the evening sits in the digestive tract through the night, fermenting and producing gas in ways that a similar meal eaten at midday would not. This does not mean eating a tiny, unsatisfying dinner — it means being thoughtful about portion size, food composition, and timing, aiming to finish eating at least two to three hours before bed where possible.

Reducing mindless evening snacking is often more impactful on bloating than any other single dietary change. Evening grazing — the habit of continuing to eat in small amounts through the hours after dinner, often while watching television or scrolling, often from processed or salty snacks — adds to the digestive load at precisely the time when the digestive system is least able to process it efficiently. It adds sodium, adds calories, and adds fermentable material to a gut that is winding down rather than gearing up. If evening snacking is a significant part of your current pattern, addressing it gradually — by eating a more satisfying dinner, by creating a clear end-of-eating time, by replacing the habit with something else that meets the emotional need it serves — tends to produce visible improvements in morning comfort quite quickly.

A gentle walk after dinner, as mentioned above, serves double duty: it supports digestion and helps gas move through the system before you lie down, and it creates a natural transition from the eating period of the evening to the winding-down period, making it psychologically easier to stop grazing and move toward rest.

Your sleep setup matters for bloating in ways that are easy to overlook. Sleeping on your left side, where anatomy is favorable, allows the large intestine to empty more effectively overnight, which can reduce the gas accumulation and digestive discomfort that contribute to morning bloating. Elevating the head of your bed slightly, if acid reflux is part of your bloating picture, can also reduce the overnight digestive disruption that translates to morning discomfort.

Creating a genuine wind-down routine — turning off screens, dimming lights, reducing mental and emotional stimulation in the hour before bed —

supports both sleep quality and digestion. When the nervous system is able to shift fully into parasympathetic mode before sleep, digestion and gut motility operate more efficiently through the night. The body that goes to sleep calm and well-regulated wakes up feeling meaningfully different from the body that falls asleep in a state of incomplete deactivation.

YOUR 7-DAY DEBLOAT RESET

Rather than a rigid protocol, this is a gentle framework for seven days focused on the habits most likely to reduce bloating visibly and quickly. It is designed to be practiced alongside the morning ritual established in Chapter 3, and to work within a real and busy life rather than requiring a perfect set of circumstances.

Each morning begins with your pink salt ritual — the warm water, the modest pinch of salt, the optional lemon, the few quiet minutes before the day begins. This is your anchor, your kept promise to yourself, the foundation on which each day is built.

Hydration through the day is the next layer — aiming for six to eight glasses of water, distributed across the waking hours, with particular attention to drinking water before meals and in the mid-afternoon window when hydration often lapses. If you currently drink very little water, an immediate dramatic increase can itself cause temporary bloating as your body adjusts, so build gradually rather than flooding your system all at once.

Meals for these seven days are built around whole, unprocessed foods as much as practically possible. Not perfectly — life does not accommodate perfection — but with a conscious shift away from packaged and processed foods and toward meals you have assembled yourself from recognizable ingredients. Protein at every meal, plenty of vegetables, fiber from a variety of sources, and the kind of moderate, satisfying portions that leave you comfortable rather than stuffed or still hungry.

After at least one meal each day — ideally dinner — take a ten-minute walk. Even a short loop around the block. Even gentle movement through the house. Something that physically activates digestion before you sit back down for the evening.

Each evening, create a clear end to eating — ideally two to three hours before bed. Notice what happens in those hours between dinner and sleep, and if grazing is a current pattern, find something to replace it: a warming herbal tea, a relaxing activity that keeps your hands occupied, a short reading practice, anything that creates a satisfying sense of closure to the eating day.

Sleep, for these seven days, is treated as a priority rather than a luxury. A consistent bedtime, a genuinely dark and cool room, a screen-free wind-down period of at least thirty minutes. Not because perfect sleep is always achievable, but because the intention to support your sleep changes the conditions you create for it.

At the end of each day, take thirty seconds to notice one thing that felt lighter, more comfortable, or more in control than it might have felt a week ago. Not a formal journal entry — just a moment of recognition. The accumulation of these small observations is the evidence of real progress, and it matters.

By day seven, many women notice genuine changes — less morning puffiness, a more comfortable midsection through the afternoon and evening, a feeling of lighter energy, clothes that fit with less variability. Some women notice these changes within the first two to three days. The timeline varies with individual physiology, current diet, stress levels, and sleep quality. What matters is not the speed but the direction.

PROGRESS BEYOND A FLAT STOMACH

There is a tendency, in wellness culture, to make a flat stomach the primary measure of success — the visual benchmark against which all other progress is evaluated. And while feeling comfortable and un-bloated in your body is a genuinely worthwhile goal that deserves to be taken seriously, it is worth ending this chapter with a broader perspective.

Feeling lighter means more than the absence of bloating. It means moving through your day with physical ease. It means clothes that feel comfortable and confidence that is not contingent on a single number or a single morning mirror check. It means a digestive system that is functioning well enough that you can eat a nourishing meal and feel good afterward rather than immediately uncomfortable.

Feeling more energized is a form of progress that no mirror can capture. Sleeping better is a form of progress. Making food choices from a place of genuine nourishment rather than frantic craving management is a form of progress. Feeling calmer and more in control of the daily cycle of eating and body experience is progress that matters deeply, even when it does not produce an immediately visible physical result.

Consistency, practiced with compassion, produces results that intensity followed by burnout never can. The woman who eats well eighty percent of the time, hydrates consistently, sleeps reasonably, and moves her body gently and regularly will feel better in six months than the woman who attempts a perfect protocol for two weeks and then abandons it. Progress is not a straight line. It accommodates imperfect days, and it builds over time in ways that are sometimes only visible when you look back over weeks rather than hours.

Your body is not your enemy. Your belly is not your enemy. It is asking for support, and you are learning to give it exactly that.

In the next chapter, we turn our attention to energy — the vitality that so many women over forty feel has quietly slipped away, and the practical, sustainable strategies for genuinely getting it back.

You are building something real here. Keep going.

5

CRUSH CRAVINGS, BOOST ENERGY, AND STOP EMOTIONAL EATING

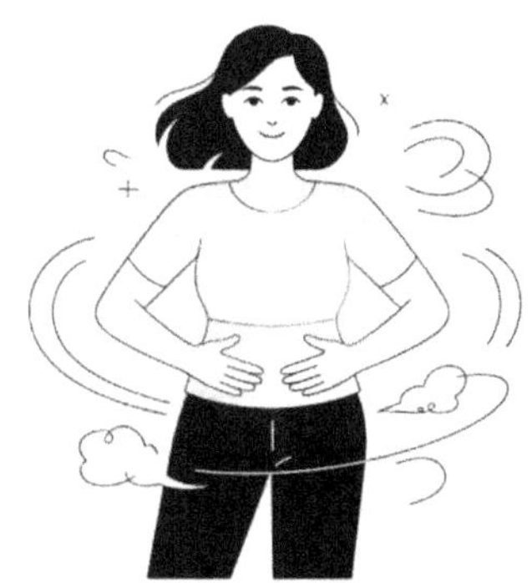

IT USUALLY HAPPENS AT THE SAME TIME EVERY DAY.

For many women, it is the mid-afternoon — somewhere between two and four o'clock, when the morning's momentum has faded and the evening still feels far away. The energy drops, the focus blurs, and from somewhere deep in the brain comes a signal that feels less like hunger and more like urgency. Something sweet. Something salty. Something that will fix the flatness of this particular moment and carry you to the other side of it.

For others, it arrives later — after dinner, when the day is technically done but the nervous system has not yet wound down, and the kitchen becomes a place of restless return. A little of this, a little of that, not because you are hungry but because something unresolved is looking for resolution in the most available place.

And then comes the familiar aftermath: the mild self-recrimination, the mental tallying of damage, the quiet resolve that tomorrow will be different. The wondering why, after years of caring about your health, after all the attempts and restarts and genuine efforts, this particular thing — food, cravings, the feeling of being out of control in the kitchen — remains so stubbornly difficult to manage.

Here is what nobody told you, and what this chapter is going to make very clear: the cravings you experience are not a character flaw. They are not evidence of weakness, or lack of discipline, or some fundamental inability to be the person you want to be around food. They are the predictable output of a specific set of biological, hormonal, and psychological conditions — conditions that have real names, real mechanisms, and real solutions that have nothing to do with trying harder.

Understanding those conditions is the beginning of genuine freedom.

WHY CRAVINGS FEEL STRONGER NOW

If your relationship with food felt more manageable in your twenties and thirties, and has become progressively more complicated since then, you are not imagining the change. The hormonal landscape of perimenopause and menopause creates specific, documented shifts in appetite regulation, reward processing, and stress response that make food cravings both more frequent and more intense for many women.

Estrogen has a direct influence on the brain's reward and pleasure systems, particularly through its interaction with dopamine — the neurotransmitter associated with motivation, pleasure, and the anticipation of reward. When estrogen levels are steady and sufficient, these systems are relatively well-regulated. As estrogen fluctuates and declines, so does some of the natural dopamine signaling that makes daily life feel rewarding and manageable without requiring external reinforcement. The result, for many women, is a subtle but persistent sense of flatness or dissatisfaction — a feeling that something is missing — that the brain learns to temporarily relieve through food, particularly foods that are dense in sugar, fat, and salt, which activate dopamine pathways powerfully and reliably.

This is not a choice. It is neurochemistry adapting to a changed hormonal environment. And once you understand it as such, the craving for a chocolate bar at three in the afternoon becomes something to address with practical strategy rather than something to feel ashamed of.

Serotonin — the neurotransmitter most associated with mood, calm, and a sense of general wellbeing — is also influenced by estrogen, and its decline contributes to the anxiety, low mood, and emotional fragility that many women experience during perimenopause. Carbohydrates, particularly simple sugars, temporarily boost serotonin production, which is why carbohydrate cravings intensify during times of hormonal fluctuation, stress, and poor sleep. Your brain is reaching for the fastest available source of neurochemical relief. It is not irrational. It is just working with an incomplete set of tools.

Cortisol — by now a familiar presence in this book — plays a central role in craving intensity. Chronic stress elevates cortisol, and elevated cortisol directly increases appetite, specifically for high-calorie, high-reward foods. This effect is evolutionary — in a survival context, stress signals a need for rapid energy, and the brain responds by driving consumption of the most energy-dense food available. In a modern context, where stress is rarely a physical survival emergency but is instead the chronic pressure of too many demands and too little rest, this drive toward food becomes a misapplied survival mechanism that produces cravings at precisely the times when your life feels most overwhelming.

Poor sleep intensifies every element of this picture. As we discussed in Chapter 1, sleep deprivation raises ghrelin and suppresses leptin — meaning you wake up hungrier, less able to feel full, and significantly more likely to choose high-calorie, high-reward foods. It also reduces activity in the prefrontal cortex — the rational, planning part of the brain — while increasing reactivity in the limbic system — the emotional, impulse-driven part. The sleep-deprived brain is, neurologically, a brain that is more likely to reach for the cookie and less capable of thinking past the craving toward a more considered choice.

And then there is the history of restriction. If you have spent years cycling through periods of strict dietary control followed by rebound overeating — which is the experience of the majority of women who have tried conventional dieting approaches — your brain has been trained in a specific way. Restriction teaches the brain that food is scarce and valuable, that the current period of abundance should be exploited before the next restriction begins, and that certain foods carry a forbidden quality that makes them neurologically more compelling than they would be if they were simply available and unremarkable. The binge-restrict cycle does not get easier with more willpower. It gets embedded deeper in the brain's operating system with every repetition, until cravings feel not just strong but genuinely unmanageable.

None of this is your fault. All of it is workable.

WILLPOWER IS NOT THE REAL PROBLEM

There is a particularly exhausting quality to the advice that women receive about cravings and food control, because it almost always circles back to the same implied message: you simply need to want it more. To be more disciplined. To care enough about your health to override the urge. To find the motivation and hold onto it.

This advice is not only unhelpful. It is scientifically inaccurate.

Willpower is a real cognitive resource, and like all cognitive resources, it is finite. Research on what psychologists call ego depletion has consistently shown that the capacity to exert self-control diminishes with use across the day — meaning that the more decisions you make, the more stress you navigate, the more demands you respond to, the less capacity you have available for the effortful override of strong impulses by late afternoon or evening. This is not weakness. It is cognitive biology operating exactly as designed.

For women over forty — who are frequently managing extensive cognitive and emotional loads, dealing with the additional neurological demands of hormonal fluctuation, often sleeping insufficiently, and carrying the accumulated fatigue of years of high performance across multiple domains — the willpower resource is typically depleted earlier and more thoroughly than in younger women or in women operating under less pressure. Asking this depleted system to override powerful, hormonally-amplified food cravings through sheer determination is like asking a battery that has been running devices all day to power something new at midnight. The capacity simply is not there, regardless of how much you care.

The solution is not more willpower. It is a smarter system — one that reduces the frequency and intensity of cravings at their source, creates environmental and habitual conditions that make better choices easier and worse choices harder, and provides genuinely effective responses to craving moments that do not rely on the depleted resource of late-day self-control.

Self-blame keeps women stuck in this cycle because it focuses attention on the wrong variable. If you believe the problem is insufficient willpower, you keep trying to generate more willpower, which keeps failing, which generates more self-blame, which adds to the stress and emotional exhaustion that deplete the system further. It is a loop that cannot be broken by turning up the intensity of the same approach.

What breaks the loop is a different approach entirely. One that begins with compassion — genuine, practical compassion, not the soft variety that excuses every choice and expects no accountability, but the kind that accurately identifies what is actually happening and responds with intelligence rather than shame.

THE AFTERNOON ENERGY CRASH

If there is one experience that most women over forty describe in nearly identical terms, it is the afternoon crash — that particular dropping away of energy and focus that arrives, reliably, at some point between two and five o'clock and makes the second half of the day feel like wading through something considerably thicker than air.

The crash is real, and it has multiple contributing causes that are almost always operating simultaneously.

Blood sugar instability is frequently at the center of it. When breakfast is skipped, or is composed primarily of simple carbohydrates without much protein or fat — a piece of toast, a bowl of cereal, a smoothie heavy on fruit — blood sugar rises quickly and then falls relatively quickly, leaving you depleted well before lunch. When lunch is similarly unbalanced, or is eaten very late, the blood sugar pattern continues its rollercoaster, and by mid-afternoon the system is depleted and demanding a rapid refuel. This demand is experienced as an intense craving for sugar or refined carbohydrates — the fastest available fuel — and the brain registers it as urgent.

Dehydration contributes significantly and is almost universally underestimated. Even mild dehydration — the kind that produces no obvious sensation of thirst — impairs cognitive function, reduces energy, and creates a fatigue that is often indistinguishable from hunger. Many women who experience a significant mid-afternoon energy drop are, at least in part, simply underhydrated from a morning of coffee and insufficient water. Drinking a large glass of water at the first sign of afternoon fatigue before reaching for food is a surprisingly effective first response.

The cortisol curve plays a natural role as well. Cortisol peaks in the early morning, providing energy and alertness, and gradually declines through the day. For most people, there is a natural energy dip in the early afternoon that corresponds to the lowest point of this cortisol arc — an entirely normal biological rhythm that has nothing to do with your choices and everything to do with your physiology. When this natural dip is compounded by blood sugar instability, dehydration, poor sleep, and a morning of high cognitive demand, it becomes the dramatic crash that sends you to the snack cabinet.

The mental and emotional load that many women carry is also a genuine energy consumer that rarely gets acknowledged as such. Decision-making, emotional management, navigating complex interpersonal dynamics, holding multiple responsibilities simultaneously — these are all cognitively expensive activities that draw on the same neurological resources as physical energy. A woman who has spent the morning managing other people's needs, navigating workplace demands, and making dozens of decisions about logistics and communication has genuinely used significant energy by afternoon — even if she has not moved very much or done anything that looks physically exhausting.

Understanding the afternoon crash as the predictable result of multiple compounding factors allows you to address it strategically rather than experiencing it as a personal failing.

EMOTIONAL EATING IN REAL LIFE

Let's talk about this honestly, because it deserves more than the oversimplified treatment it usually receives.

Emotional eating — eating in response to feelings rather than physical hunger — is not a disorder, and it is not something that only affects people who lack discipline or self-awareness. It is a deeply human behavior that develops because food genuinely does provide emotional relief, at least in the short term. It activates pleasure pathways in the brain. It provides a sensory experience that temporarily interrupts difficult emotions. It offers comfort in the immediate moment in a way that is reliable, accessible, and requires no particular effort.

For women over forty, emotional eating is often woven into the fabric of daily life in ways that have accumulated over years. The piece of chocolate that marks the end of a stressful workday. The bowl of something satisfying eaten in front of the television after everyone else's needs have been met and you finally have twenty minutes to yourself. The extra helpings at dinner after a day when you felt unseen or underappreciated. The kitchen grazing that begins not from hunger but from a kind of restless searching — for comfort, for reward, for a moment of pleasure in a day that has contained too little of it.

None of these behaviors are signs of weakness. They are signs of a life that is, in various ways, not meeting certain needs — for rest, for pleasure, for emotional acknowledgment, for reward, for relief from the constant demands of caring for everyone else. Food fills those gaps temporarily because it is available and immediate and because it works, in the short term, to provide what the moment is lacking.

The problem is not that food provides comfort — it is a legitimate source of pleasure and should be. The problem is when food becomes the only available source of comfort, relief, or reward, and when the reliance on it for emotional regulation becomes a source of shame, physical discomfort, and disconnection from your body's actual hunger and satiety signals.

Reward eating — the deeply entrenched cultural habit of treating food as the primary reward for effort, stress, and achievement — is something that most women over forty learned before they had any conscious awareness of learning it. It is written into the fabric of how most families and cultures relate to celebration, comfort, and difficulty. Recognizing it as a learned pattern rather than an innate weakness is the first step toward choosing, gradually and without drama, whether it serves you.

Stress snacking — particularly the evening kind, where hands and mouths move automatically while eyes are on a screen and the day's tensions remain unprocessed — is often not about hunger at all. It is about the nervous system seeking stimulation, or the body seeking to complete the stress cycle that the day has opened. Addressing the underlying stress, in whatever form is accessible — a short walk, a few minutes of deliberate breathing, a bath, a conversation, putting a blanket over your lap and genuinely resting rather than grazing — often dissolves the snacking impulse without requiring any direct engagement with the food itself.

Loneliness eating, which is rarely named but is deeply common, especially for women in midlife who may be navigating shifts in relationships, identity, and social connection alongside the physical changes of hormonal transition, deserves particular compassion. Food is company of a kind. It fills space and silence in ways that feel soothing. Acknowledging this honestly — without judgment, simply as an observation about what a particular eating moment is actually about — opens the door to addressing the real need rather than temporarily managing its symptom.

BUILD MEALS THAT REDUCE CRAVINGS

The most reliable way to reduce food cravings is not to white-knuckle your way through them. It is to build your meals in a way that prevents the blood sugar instability, nutritional insufficiency, and sustained hunger that generate cravings in the first place.

Protein is the most important piece of this picture, and it is the nutrient that is most commonly insufficient in the diets of women who experience frequent and intense cravings. Protein digests slowly, which means it sustains blood sugar stability and promotes genuine satiety for several hours after a meal. It stimulates the release of satiety hormones — peptide YY, GLP-1 — that communicate fullness to the brain. And it supports muscle maintenance, which matters enormously for metabolic health after forty.

Including a meaningful amount of protein at every meal — particularly at breakfast, which sets the blood sugar and hunger tone for the hours that follow — is one of the single most impactful dietary changes a woman over forty can make for craving management. Eggs, Greek yogurt, cottage cheese, smoked salmon, leftover chicken or turkey, legumes — the sources matter less than the consistency. A breakfast containing twenty to thirty grams of protein will carry you to lunch in a meaningfully different hormonal and metabolic state than a breakfast consisting primarily of toast or cereal or fruit alone.

Fiber works alongside protein to support sustained satiety and stable blood sugar. Vegetables, legumes, whole grains, nuts, seeds, and fruit all provide fiber in different forms, and including a variety across meals creates the kind of digestive steadiness that prevents the sharp blood sugar fluctuations that trigger intense cravings. The key is consistency and variety rather than any specific target number.

Healthy fats — from avocado, olive oil, nuts, seeds, fatty fish — are the third component of a genuinely satisfying meal. Fat slows digestion, contributes to satiety, and provides the raw material for hormone production that becomes particularly important during perimenopause and menopause. Meals that are very low in fat, regardless of their caloric content, tend to produce less sustained satisfaction, which leaves the brain searching for the missing component in the hours that follow.

The architecture of your eating through the day matters as much as any individual meal. Regular meals at consistent times, with protein, fiber, and fat represented at each one, create a metabolic rhythm that keeps blood sugar stable, keeps hunger hormones in a manageable range, and dramatically reduces the intensity and frequency of the urgent, specific cravings that drive most dietary derailment. Skipping meals, eating irregularly, or going very long periods between eating all create the blood sugar and hunger conditions that make cravings feel unmanageable.

Snacks, when needed, are most effective when they follow the same principles as meals in miniature. A small portion of protein and fat together — a few nuts and a piece of cheese, some hummus with vegetables, a hard-boiled egg, Greek yogurt with a few berries — provides the bridge between meals that a handful of crackers or a piece of fruit alone cannot sustain.

QUICK ENERGY BOOSTERS THAT ACTUALLY HELP

When the afternoon crash arrives, the instinct is to reach for caffeine or sugar — two things that provide a brief lift followed by a deeper descent, compounding the very problem you were trying to solve. Here are the strategies that actually support genuine, sustained energy without the crash.

Morning light is the most underused energy tool available to most people. Exposure to natural light in the first thirty to sixty minutes after waking sets your circadian rhythm, regulates your cortisol awakening response, and communicates to your brain what time of day it is in a way that supports better energy distribution across the whole day. A ten-minute walk outside, or simply sitting near a bright window with your morning ritual water, creates a biological foundation for better daytime energy that no supplement can replicate.

Hydration remains relevant throughout the day, not just in the morning. The mid-afternoon fatigue that sends many women to the snack cupboard is frequently, at least in part, dehydration. Drinking a large glass of water at the first sign of afternoon energy dropping — before making any food choices — is a thirty-second intervention that resolves the issue entirely for a surprising number of women.

A short walk in the early afternoon — even five to ten minutes — is one of the most effective known interventions for the post-lunch energy dip. It stimulates circulation, delivers oxygenated blood to the brain, activates the muscles and nervous system, and has been shown in research to improve both energy and cognitive performance in the hours that follow. It requires no equipment, no preparation, and no particular motivation — just the willingness to step away from the desk or the house for a few minutes at the moment when doing so feels least appealing.

Protein-rich meals — as discussed above — provide the kind of sustained energy that caffeine simulates but cannot genuinely replace. A lunch that is built around a substantial protein source, with vegetables and some healthy fat, will carry you through the afternoon in a fundamentally different metabolic state than a lunch that is heavy in refined carbohydrates and light in protein.

Brief stretch breaks throughout the day — even two or three minutes of standing up, rolling your shoulders, folding forward, and taking a few deep breaths — interrupt the physical and neurological stagnation of prolonged sitting and provide a genuine micro-reset that improves both energy and mood. The physiological benefits are real, and the interruption of sedentary patterns also reduces the muscle stiffness and tension that accumulate across a day of desk work and contribute to afternoon fatigue.

Breath resets — deliberate, slow, deep breathing for sixty to ninety seconds — activate the parasympathetic nervous system and produce a measurable reduction in cortisol and physical tension. The box breathing pattern — inhaling for four counts, holding for four, exhaling for four, holding for four — is simple, requires no special skill, and produces effects that are immediate and genuine.

THE CRAVING RESCUE PLAN

Every woman who has successfully navigated the terrain of food cravings long-term has some version of what we might call a rescue plan — a set of practiced responses for the moments when a craving arrives with force and the depleted willpower system is not available to simply override it.

Here is a practical sequence to practice until it becomes automatic.

The first step is the pause. Not a long deliberation — just a ten-second interruption between the craving signal and any action. During that ten seconds, you are simply noticing: a craving has arrived. It is a feeling, not an emergency. Nothing terrible will happen if it is not immediately resolved.

The second step is hydration. A full glass of water, drunk slowly. This addresses the dehydration component of many cravings, introduces a one-to-two-minute gap between impulse and action, and occasionally — more often than you might expect — resolves the craving entirely.

If the craving persists, the third step is to name what you actually need. Not what you want to eat — what you are actually experiencing. Tired? Stressed? Bored? Lonely? Seeking reward? Trying to avoid something? This naming is not a judgment. It is information. And occasionally, simply naming the actual need is enough to allow a different response to it — a rest, a brief walk, a connection with someone, a moment of acknowledged achievement.

The ten-minute delay is the fourth tool. If you still want to eat something after the pause, the water, and the naming, decide to wait ten minutes before acting. In behavioral terms, this delay dramatically reduces the likelihood of acting on an impulse, because the urgency of most craving signals diminishes significantly within ten minutes if it is not immediately fed. Set a timer if it helps. Do something else during those ten minutes — move, breathe, change location.

Changing your environment briefly is one of the most underrated craving interruption strategies. If you are in the kitchen when the craving arrives, leave the kitchen. If you are sitting, stand up and move to a different room. The environmental cue and the craving are often linked, and removing yourself from the cue physically weakens the craving signal meaningfully.

If, after all of this, you genuinely want to eat something, eat intentionally. Portion out a specific amount of whatever you are choosing, sit down with it away from screens, eat it slowly and with full attention, and experience it as a deliberate choice rather than a reactive consumption. Food eaten this way, with consciousness and genuine enjoyment, provides far more satisfaction than the same food eaten quickly and guiltily, and it does not feed the shame cycle that keeps emotional eating patterns entrenched.

HOW TO BOUNCE BACK AFTER A BAD DAY

There will be days when none of this works perfectly. Days when the craving wins entirely, when the evening spirals into grazing that you did not intend, when a difficult day or a terrible night's sleep or a moment of genuine emotional pain leads you to food in ways that leave you feeling worse rather than better.

These days are not failures. They are human.

Here is the single most important thing to understand about an off-plan meal, an emotional eating episode, a night of unintended kitchen grazing: it changes nothing about your overall trajectory unless you allow the story you tell about it to change everything. One imperfect evening does not undo a week of genuine progress. One day of poor choices does not reset the metabolic, hormonal, and habitual foundations you have been building. The damage done by the food is almost always significantly less than the damage done by the shame and self-criticism that follow it.

Guilt, in the context of eating, is not a protective or corrective emotion. It does not prevent repetition of the behavior. What it reliably does is elevate cortisol, which activates the very craving mechanisms you are trying to manage, and erodes the sense of self-efficacy that makes future good choices feel possible. The woman who eats something she regrets and then immediately decides she has failed and might as well continue — the "I've blown it now, so I'll start fresh Monday" internal logic — is not experiencing a crisis of willpower. She is experiencing the predictable neurological effects of shame in a stress-response system that copes with distress through the most available source of relief.

Recovery does not begin on Monday. It does not require a declaration or a new plan or an erasing of what happened. It begins at the very next choice. Dinner went sideways. The next choice — the glass of water before bed, the morning ritual tomorrow, breakfast made with intention — is recovery. Not redemption, not compensation, not starting over. Simply continuing, from the very next moment, with the same care and consistency that characterized the days before the difficult one.

The women who succeed long-term at any wellness approach are not the ones who never have bad days. They are the ones who have developed the skill of returning — quietly, without drama, without the theatrical restart — to their practices, their rituals, their general direction, immediately after a disruption. That skill of returning is built through practice, and it is built most reliably by removing the judgment and shame that make returning feel complicated and delayed.

You had a hard day. Today is different. Drink your water.

BECOMING A WOMAN WHO TRUSTS HERSELF AGAIN

There is a version of you that exists beyond the craving cycles, beyond the afternoon crashes, beyond the emotional eating episodes and the morning-after recriminations. A version who eats in a way that feels natural and nourishing rather than fraught and complicated. Who moves through most days with steady, adequate energy rather than swinging between highs and crashes. Who experiences food as one genuine source of pleasure among many, rather than as the primary available source of relief and reward.

This is not an idealized fantasy. It is a genuinely achievable state, built not through some dramatic transformation but through the accumulation of the small, consistent practices this book is helping you establish.

Trust in yourself around food is not something you either have or do not have. It is something you build, one kept promise at a time. When you follow through on the morning ritual, you build it. When you choose a balanced lunch instead of skipping it and then crashing later, you build it. When you pause before a craving and give yourself the ten minutes, and the craving passes, and you do not eat the thing, you build it. And when you do eat the thing — intentionally, with pleasure, without shame — and then return to your practice the next morning without drama, you build it in a different but equally important way.

The relationship you are developing with your body in this process is one of the most significant shifts this entire reset is designed to create. Not a relationship of control and punishment, but one of genuine attunement — learning to hear what your body is actually communicating, to distinguish between physical hunger and emotional hunger, to respond to real needs rather than managing symptoms, and to make choices that leave you feeling better rather than worse in the hours and days that follow.

Energy that is stable and genuine. Cravings that are manageable rather than overwhelming. A sense of being in control of your choices rather than controlled by them. These are not the destination of a perfect diet. They are the natural outcome of a body that is being consistently nourished, rested, hydrated, and supported — a body whose stress load is being thoughtfully managed, whose mornings begin with intention, whose meals provide genuine sustenance rather than blood sugar chaos.

You are building that body. Not by being perfect, but by being consistent. Not by eliminating every difficult moment, but by responding to difficult moments with an expanding toolkit rather than a depleting one.

In the next chapter, we turn to one of the most fundamental elements of the entire reset — sleep. Because everything we have discussed in these pages becomes easier, more effective, and more sustainable when you are genuinely rested. And for women over forty, reclaiming the quality of your sleep may be the single highest-return investment you can make in your overall wellbeing.

You are not the woman who starts over every Monday. You are the woman who simply keeps going.

6

LET'S TALK ABOUT SOMETHING THAT ALMOST NO ONE TALKS ABOUT HONESTLY.

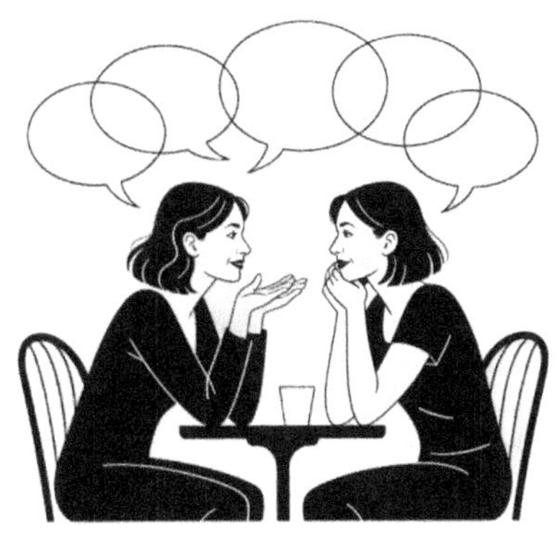

LET'S TALK

It is ten at night. The house is quiet. You have done everything right today. You drank your water in the morning. You ate a sensible breakfast. You made good choices at lunch. You skipped the cookies someone brought to the office. You had a reasonable dinner. And now here you are, standing in front of the pantry, reaching for something you promised yourself you would not eat. Maybe it is cookies. Maybe it is chips. Maybe it is a handful of chocolate that turns into three handfuls. Maybe it is ice cream straight from the container.

And as you eat it, part of you is already ashamed. Another part of you is saying, *why does this always happen?* A third part of you is vaguely angry, at yourself, at your body, at the whole frustrating situation. By the time you finally put the food away and head to bed, you feel defeated, bloated, and a little lonely. You tell yourself that tomorrow will be different.

Tomorrow you will try harder. Tomorrow you will have more willpower. Tomorrow will be the real beginning.

But tomorrow comes, and at some point, usually in the afternoon or evening, the same scene repeats. Maybe not with exactly the same food. Maybe not in exactly the same spot. But the pattern is painfully familiar. And over weeks, months, and years, this pattern quietly becomes one of the most painful parts of being a woman over forty. It is not the cravings themselves that hurt most. It is the feeling that you cannot trust yourself around food anymore. That you have lost something you used to have. That no matter how determined you are in the morning, the evening version of you will find a way to undo it.

I want you to know something, right up front, before we go any further. You are not broken. You are not weak. You are not a woman with a willpower problem. Your cravings are not a character flaw, and your emotional eating is not evidence that something is deeply wrong with you. Every single woman who has struggled with this struggle is struggling with something real, understandable, and absolutely addressable, once she understands what is actually going on.

This chapter is going to give you that understanding, and it is going to give you tools. Not fantasy tools. Not willpower tools. Real, practical, gentle tools that work in the kitchen, in the office, at the pantry door, and in the evening, when the day has been long and the cravings are loud. By the time you finish this chapter, you are going to know why this keeps happening, and you are going to have a set of responses that actually match your life.

Why Cravings Feel Stronger Now

The first thing to understand is that the cravings you are experiencing now are not the same cravings you had in your twenties or thirties. They may look similar from the outside, but underneath, they are being driven by a different set of forces.

Cravings in midlife are amplified by hormonal shifts. As estrogen levels fluctuate and then decline, your brain's sensitivity to serotonin, the feel-good chemical, changes. When serotonin dips, your brain often looks for something to boost it, and one of the fastest ways to get a temporary serotonin lift is through sugar and refined carbohydrates. This is not your imagination. Your brain is literally asking for these foods as a form of self-medication when your hormonal chemistry is unsettled.

Progesterone, which has a calming effect on your nervous system, also declines in this season of life. When progesterone is lower, your nervous system feels more agitated and less at ease. Food, especially sweet and carb-rich food, provides a quick, if temporary, sense of calm. You are not reaching for the cookies because you are weak. You are reaching for them because your body is seeking a regulating agent, and the cookies provide one, at least for a few minutes.

Then there is cortisol. When cortisol is elevated for extended periods, as it often is for women juggling careers, families, aging parents, and everything else, it triggers cravings for sugar and simple carbohydrates. Cortisol is essentially saying, *this is hard, we need quick energy to get through it*. And quick energy, in modern life, means sweet, starchy, or processed food.

On top of all of this, midlife often comes with poor sleep. Hormonal shifts disrupt sleep quality. Stress keeps your mind racing at three in the morning. Hot flashes wake you up. And when you wake up tired, your hunger hormones shift dramatically. One hormone, called ghrelin, rises when you are underslept, making you physically hungrier all day. Another, called leptin, decreases, making it harder to feel satisfied by the food you eat. You wake up hungrier, stay hungrier, and crave more intensely, all because of a few hours of missed sleep.

Add in the long history of restrictive dieting that most women over forty are carrying. Years, sometimes decades, of cutting foods, skipping meals, following rigid plans, and suppressing hunger. Your body remembers all of this. When you have spent years restricting, your nervous system stays on alert for the next restriction, and any time it senses one coming, it drives you toward food more forcefully, just in case. This is not weakness. This is a body trying to protect you from deprivation it has learned to fear.

And then there is emotional exhaustion, which we will talk about more shortly. By midlife, many women are carrying an invisible load that would crush almost anyone. Work, family, aging parents, financial worries, marriage questions, identity shifts, all of it piled on top of a body that is changing. Food often becomes the one accessible source of comfort in a life that rarely offers enough of it.

Finally, blood sugar plays a massive role. When your meals do not keep your blood sugar steady, you end up on a rollercoaster of highs and lows. Every dip triggers cravings. Every spike leads to another dip. You can be on this rollercoaster all day without realizing it, and by evening, you are a passenger who has been flung around for twelve hours. No wonder the pantry calls. Your blood sugar is begging for something fast.

So please hear this clearly. Your cravings are not random. They are not proof of weakness. They are the predictable result of hormones, stress, sleep, history, emotion, and blood sugar, all interacting in a body that is doing its best. Once you see them this way, you can stop blaming yourself and start responding wisely.

Willpower Is Not the Real Problem

There is a story we have all been told about food. That some people have willpower and some people do not. That the people who are fit and healthy are the ones with better discipline. That if you could just want it more, try harder, and resist better, you would succeed.

This story is wrong, and it has been harming women for decades.

The truth is that willpower is a finite, unreliable resource. It is at its highest in the morning, after a good night's sleep, with a calm schedule, a full stomach, and low stress. It drops throughout the day as you make decisions, handle stress, and spend energy. By evening, after a long day of work, family demands, and the thousand small decisions that make up adult life, your willpower is nearly empty. That is not a character flaw. That is biology.

This is why you can be so strong in the morning and so vulnerable in the evening. It is not because the morning version of you is the real you and the evening version is somehow fake. It is because the evening version of you is depleted. She does not need more willpower. She needs a different environment, a different plan, and a different relationship with the whole situation.

When you rely on willpower to control your eating, you are essentially trying to white-knuckle your way through each day, using up a resource that runs out faster than the day lasts. Every time you resist a craving through force, you deplete your willpower a little more. By the time you get to the real challenges of the day, your willpower tank is empty, and the cravings win.

The women who succeed with food in midlife are not women with super-human willpower. They are women who have stopped relying on willpower entirely. They have built systems around themselves that make good choices easier and poor choices less automatic. They have set up their kitchens so the foods that trigger them are not constantly within reach. They have planned their meals so they are not making high-stakes decisions at eight in the evening while tired. They have routines that bring calm instead of chaos. They have reduced the number of times per day they need to rely on willpower at all, because they have designed their environment to support them.

This is the reframe that changes everything. You are not failing because you lack willpower. You are failing because willpower is the wrong tool for the job. Smart systems beat hard effort, every time.

What does this look like in practice? It looks like keeping the foods that trigger nightly binges out of the house entirely, not as punishment, but as kindness to your evening self. It looks like planning your meals ahead so that dinner is almost automatic instead of a decision you make while exhausted. It looks like building a morning ritual you do not have to think about. It looks like going to bed earlier so your hormones support you instead of sabotaging you. It looks like saying yes to help, delegating, setting limits, so the stress on your nervous system is not maxed out.

Every system you build is one less moment where you have to rely on willpower. And over time, as these systems accumulate, the cravings quiet down, because you are no longer running on empty.

You are not a woman who needs more discipline. You are a woman who needs a better setup. Those are very different things.

The Afternoon Energy Crash

Let's talk about that three in the afternoon moment, because almost every woman reading this knows it intimately.

You were fine in the morning. You got through lunch. And then, somewhere between two and four in the afternoon, something shifts. Your brain goes foggy. Your body gets heavy. Your motivation disappears. You find yourself reading the same email three times. You feel like you need a nap, or a coffee, or something sweet. Nothing else on the to-do list feels doable, and you are still hours away from being off work or off duty.

This afternoon crash is one of the most common experiences of midlife, and it has multiple causes, most of which are fixable.

Skipping breakfast or eating a breakfast that does not sustain you is a major contributor. When your morning meal is too light, too carb-heavy, or missing protein, your blood sugar spikes and crashes within a couple of hours. By the time lunch arrives, you are already running on fumes. Lunch picks you up briefly, but if it too is unbalanced, the same pattern repeats, and the afternoon crash is essentially inevitable.

Poor sleep from the night before shows up in the afternoon with striking reliability. If you did not sleep well, your body will find a way to demand rest around mid-afternoon, whether you have time for it or not. This is the body trying to catch up on something it did not get at night. It is not laziness. It is biology asserting itself.

Chronic stress drains your energy throughout the day, often in hidden ways. Your nervous system is working overtime to keep up, and by mid-afternoon, it is tapped out. The mental load of caring for everyone, remembering everything, and managing everything takes a toll that is easy to underestimate.

Dehydration is a sneaky culprit. By three in the afternoon, many women have had coffee, maybe a glass of water with lunch, and nothing else. Your body has been running on partial hydration for hours. Mild dehydration reduces energy, focus, and mood, and mimics hunger, which is why many afternoon cravings are actually thirst in disguise.

Unbalanced meals, as I mentioned, keep your blood sugar rollercoaster moving all day. If lunch was mostly carbs with very little protein or fat, expect a crash. If lunch was too small, expect a crash. If lunch was rushed and eaten at your desk while you kept working, your body did not get the signal that a meal had happened, and the crash comes anyway.

And decision fatigue, the mental exhaustion of making hundreds of small choices throughout the day, compounds everything. By afternoon, your brain is tired. And a tired brain reaches for easy dopamine hits, usually in the form of sugar or caffeine.

The solution is not more coffee, though we will get to the role caffeine plays. The solution is to eat meals that keep your blood sugar steady, stay hydrated throughout the day, protect your sleep at night, and reduce the number of unnecessary decisions you are making. When these pieces come together, the afternoon crash fades, often dramatically. Many women report that within a few weeks of balancing their meals and sleeping better, the three o'clock wall they had been hitting for years simply disappears.

Emotional Eating in Real Life

Now let's sit with this one honestly, because emotional eating is one of the most misunderstood parts of a woman's relationship with food. And I want you to know, before we go any further, that I am not going to shame you about it. Emotional eating is not a disease. It is not a disorder unique to women with problems. It is, in some form, nearly universal, and it deserves to be understood with compassion rather than condemnation.

You eat for comfort sometimes. Who does not? When something hard happens, a difficult conversation, a disappointment, a worry, food can be a quiet companion. A warm bowl of something familiar feels like a hug from the inside. This is not a pathology. This is a very human response to distress, and there is no reason to be ashamed of it.

You eat for reward sometimes. After a hard day, after finishing a big project, after getting through something you dreaded, food is a celebration. A glass of wine, a piece of cake, a favorite meal. Reward eating is woven into culture for a reason. It acknowledges effort, marks moments, and brings pleasure.

You eat when you are stressed. Stress eating is one of the most common patterns among women juggling too much. When you feel overwhelmed, food becomes a moment of control, a small pleasure in a life that feels demanding. The hand reaches for the snack drawer almost automatically. Before you have decided to eat, you are already eating.

You eat out of loneliness. This one is harder to talk about, but it is real. When the house is quiet and the evening feels long, food can fill a space that human connection would fill in a different season of life. A snack while watching television can be a way of keeping yourself company.

You eat out of habit. The bowl of popcorn every night because that is what you do while watching your show. The snack at your desk every afternoon because it is where you are when the craving comes. The dessert after dinner every evening because dinner always ends with dessert. These patterns are not about hunger. They are about grooves in your life that have worn deep over time.

You eat in *I deserve this* moments. After a long week, after putting everyone else's needs first, after carrying too much, there is a voice that says, *I have earned this*. And you eat, not because your body is hungry, but because some part of you wants to give yourself something, anything, that feels like care.

I want to tell you something about all of these patterns. They are not stupid. They are not pathetic. They are the creative, often desperate attempts of a tired woman to give herself what she needs when the life she is living does not give her enough of it. Comfort. Reward. Relief. Connection. Pleasure. Permission. These are real needs. Food is just the fastest, cheapest, most accessible way to touch them briefly.

The work, then, is not to banish emotional eating. That is not possible, and the attempt will only make you feel worse. The work is to start meeting those needs in other ways, gently, over time, so that food is not the only source of comfort, reward, relief, connection, pleasure, or permission in your life. As you build those other sources, emotional eating quiets down on its own. Not because you forced it to. Because you stopped needing it as much.

This is slow work, and it is deep work, and it is worth every minute. For now, please hold this truth. Emotional eating is not proof that something is wrong with you. It is proof that something inside you is asking for care. Learning to give yourself that care is one of the most important projects of your midlife.

Build Meals That Reduce Cravings

Let's get practical now, because nothing quiets cravings like actually being well-fed.

The single most powerful food strategy for reducing cravings is building meals that keep your blood sugar steady. This sounds technical, but it is actually simple. Steady blood sugar means fewer crashes, fewer cravings, steadier energy, and a calmer relationship with food. The formula is straightforward, and you can apply it at every meal.

Start with protein. Most women over forty are under-eating protein, and it is one of the quiet reasons they are constantly hungry and craving. Every meal should contain a meaningful portion of protein. Eggs. Chicken. Fish. Yogurt. Cottage cheese. Beans. Lentils. Tofu. Good quality meat. A palm-sized portion at minimum. Protein fills you up, stabilizes blood sugar, and supports muscle, which becomes more important each year.

Add fiber. Fiber comes primarily from vegetables, fruits, beans, and whole grains. Fiber slows digestion, which keeps you fuller longer and prevents the blood sugar spikes that drive cravings. Vegetables at every meal is one of the simplest, most transformative habits you can build. Fill half your plate with vegetables whenever possible.

Include healthy fats. Fat has been demonized for decades, but in reasonable amounts, it is one of your best allies against cravings. Avocado, olive oil, nuts, seeds, eggs, fatty fish, and quality dairy all provide fats that keep you satisfied and support hormone health. Do not fear fat. Embrace it in sensible portions.

Be careful with refined carbohydrates. These are the breads, pastries, crackers, cereals, sweets, and processed snacks that cause the biggest blood sugar swings. They taste wonderful, and you do not have to banish them, but they should not be the foundation of most of your meals. When you do eat them, pair them with protein, fat, and fiber to soften their effect.

Breakfast deserves special attention because it sets the tone for the whole day. A breakfast that is mostly sugar or refined carbs, like sugary cereal, pastries, or a bagel alone, sends your blood sugar up and then crashing down, which creates craving patterns that last for hours. A breakfast with protein, fiber, and some fat, like eggs with vegetables, Greek yogurt with berries and nuts, or oatmeal with protein powder and seeds, sets a completely different trajectory. Many women who have struggled with cravings for years find that simply changing breakfast changes everything.

Snacks, when you want them, should follow the same principle. Instead of crackers alone, crackers with cheese and some vegetables. Instead of fruit alone, fruit with a handful of nuts. Instead of a granola bar, a small meal-like snack with protein. The goal is to feed your body real food that satisfies rather than just filling time.

Regular meal timing also helps. Chaos eating, where you skip meals for hours and then overeat later, creates the biggest blood sugar swings and the most intense cravings. Aim for three meaningful meals a day, spaced reasonably, with small snacks only if you are genuinely hungry between them.

You do not need to become an expert nutritionist. You just need to build plates that have protein, vegetables, healthy fats, and a reasonable amount of carbs, eaten at regular times. Within a week of doing this consistently, most women notice their cravings drop significantly. Not because they developed willpower. Because their bodies are finally satisfied.

Quick Energy Boosters That Actually Help

When your energy is low, you need tools that work quickly without creating new problems. Here are the ones that actually help.

Morning light is underused and surprisingly powerful. Get some natural light in your eyes within the first hour of waking, even if you only stand at a window or step outside for a minute. Morning light sets your body clock, improves mood, and helps your energy rise and fall more naturally through the day. It also supports better sleep that night, which supports better energy the next day. This is a gentle compounding effect that many women never experience because they go from bed to phone to coffee to car to office without ever seeing the sky.

Hydration is the quickest energy fix most women underestimate. When you feel tired mid-morning or mid-afternoon, try drinking a full glass of water before reaching for coffee or a snack. If your energy comes back within ten or fifteen minutes, you were thirsty, not tired.

Short walks are remarkable energy tools. A ten-minute walk, especially outside, does more for flagging afternoon energy than a second cup of coffee. It raises circulation, breaks mental fatigue, and resets your nervous system. If you only take one action from this chapter, adding a short walk to your afternoon could be the one that changes your days.

Protein-rich meals, as we discussed, support steady energy throughout the day. Women who eat enough protein at breakfast and lunch experience far fewer afternoon crashes than women who do not.

Stretch breaks matter more than you might expect. Sitting for hours slows circulation, stiffens your body, and contributes to mental fatigue. A few minutes of standing, stretching, or gentle movement every hour or two keeps your energy more stable than trying to power through.

Breath resets are tiny but potent. Five slow, deep breaths can shift your nervous system in under a minute. Try inhaling through your nose for four counts, holding briefly, and exhaling through your mouth for six counts. Do this five times. Your brain will clear, your shoulders will drop, and your energy will often come back.

Better sleep habits, which we will talk about in more detail soon, are the foundation underneath all of this. You cannot caffeinate your way out of chronic poor sleep. You can only rest your way out of it.

And reducing all-or-nothing thinking gives you energy you did not know you had. When you stop treating every small mistake as a catastrophe, when you stop spending mental energy on guilt and shame about what you ate or did not do, when you allow for imperfection without spiraling, you free up an enormous amount of mental bandwidth. That bandwidth translates directly into energy for the things that matter.

The Craving Rescue Plan

Now, for the moment that really matters. The moment the craving hits. The moment you are standing in front of the pantry or reaching for the snack drawer, and you can feel the pull. Here is what to do, step by step.

First, pause. Before you reach for the food, take a single breath. Just one. This tiny pause interrupts the automatic reach and gives you a moment of choice. You are not saying no yet. You are just creating a small gap between the urge and the action.

Second, drink water. Pour a glass, and drink it slowly. Many cravings are partly dehydration. Many more have a nervous system component that gets calmed by the act of pausing to drink. Sometimes the craving fades within minutes. Sometimes it does not. Either way, the water does not hurt.

Third, ask yourself a single question. *What do I actually need right now?* Not to shame yourself, not to guilt yourself out of eating, just to check in honestly.

Are you physically hungry, or are you stressed, tired, lonely, bored, or stuck? Sometimes the answer is yes, you are actually hungry, and a balanced snack is the right response. Other times, the answer is something deeper, and food will not solve it.

Fourth, if you are physically hungry, eat something with protein and substance. Not the quickest, emptiest snack. Something that will actually satisfy you. A small handful of nuts and cheese. A yogurt. A hard boiled egg. An apple with peanut butter. Something real. This kind of snack ends a craving. A tiny bag of chips often does not, because your body was asking for nourishment, not fillers.

Fifth, if you are not physically hungry, try a short delay. Tell yourself, *I will wait ten minutes before eating*. Set a timer if you need to. Many cravings dissolve on their own within ten or fifteen minutes if you simply ride them out doing something else. Go for a short walk. Call a friend. Take a shower. Get out of the kitchen. The craving is a wave, and waves break. You do not have to surf every one of them to shore.

Sixth, change your environment. A lot of emotional eating happens in the same physical locations. The couch. The pantry. The desk. If you can physically move somewhere else, even for a few minutes, the pull often loosens. Step outside. Go to a different room. Sit in your car for a moment. The location change breaks the pattern.

Seventh, if the craving is winning, and sometimes it will, eat the thing you want with intention. Put it on a plate. Sit down. Actually taste it. Enjoy it. This is very different from mindlessly eating straight from the container while standing in the kitchen or lying on the couch. Mindless eating is emotionally unsatisfying even when the food is delicious. Intentional eating, even of the same food, is usually enough to end the craving cycle instead of fueling it. You get the pleasure. You do not get the shame. You stop when you are actually satisfied.

This seven-step rescue plan is not about being perfect. It is about having something to reach for other than the food itself when the craving hits. Even doing one or two of these steps, instead of none, will often change the outcome. Over time, as these responses become more automatic, the cravings themselves grow quieter, because your nervous system learns that they no longer get instant, automatic obedience. You are, gently, rewriting the pattern.

How to Bounce Back After a Bad Day

Every woman reading this has had days where nothing goes the way she hoped. You ate more than you wanted. You gave in to the craving. You had a night of eating that felt out of control. The next morning, you wake up feeling bloated, disappointed, and tempted to write the whole week off.

I want to tell you something that, if you take it to heart, will change your relationship with food forever.

One off-plan meal changes nothing. One night of overeating does not erase your progress. One emotional evening does not undo the work you have been doing. Your body does not remember a single night the way you do, and real progress is not destroyed by single moments.

What does damage progress is what happens next. Not the meal itself, but the story you tell yourself about the meal, and what you do in the days afterward. If you wake up the next morning, take a breath, return to your morning ritual, drink your water, and make the next choice a kind one, you are still exactly on track. Nothing has been lost. You are simply continuing.

But if you wake up and decide that you have ruined it, that you have failed, that there is no point now, and you proceed to eat poorly for the rest of the day, the weekend, or the week, because you might as well, that is what causes real damage. Not the food. The spiral around the food. The guilt that leads to more eating. The shame that leads to giving up. The story that one mistake proves you cannot do this.

Resilient women know something that women caught in cycles do not. They know that recovery starts at the very next choice. Not on Monday. Not next week. Not after one more indulgence. The very next choice. The next glass of water. The next meal. The next breath.

When you can treat yourself the way you would treat a friend who had a hard night, with patience and perspective, you become unstoppable in this work. Because nothing can derail you anymore. Bad nights happen. Hard weeks happen. Life happens. And each time, you simply return, gently, to the practice. You do not have to be perfect to make real progress. You only have to keep coming back.

Guilt is not a tool for change. It masquerades as one, but it is not. Guilt depletes you. It darkens your mood. It makes the next choice harder, not easier. It keeps you stuck in the same patterns you are trying to leave. Kindness is the actual tool for change. Kindness gets you back to the ritual, back to the water, back to the balanced meal, back to the walk. Kindness does not care about perfection. Kindness cares about you.

So when the bad day comes, and it will, meet yourself with kindness. Drink a glass of water. Do the morning ritual. Go for a walk. Make a real meal. Keep going. The woman you are building is not the woman who never falls. She is the woman who always comes back.

Becoming a Woman Who Trusts Herself Again

Here is where all of this is heading, and it is worth naming clearly, because the destination is beautiful.

Every time you pause before reaching for the craving food, every time you drink water before a snack, every time you eat a balanced breakfast, every time you take a walk in the afternoon instead of a second coffee, every time you come back gently after a difficult night, you are building something much bigger than weight loss. You are building a relationship with yourself that has been strained for years, maybe decades.

You are becoming a woman who trusts herself with food. A woman whose energy feels steadier. A woman who can sit through a craving without panicking. A woman who knows the difference between real hunger and emotional noise. A woman who can enjoy a piece of cake without turning it into a crisis. A woman who keeps the small promises she makes to herself, most of the time, and forgives herself on the days she does not.

This is a transformation that runs deeper than any scale. It changes how you walk into rooms, how you feel in your body at social events, how you handle stress, how you respond to challenges in every area of your life. When you trust yourself around food, you start trusting yourself in other places too. You become steadier. You become more confident. You become more yourself.

None of this happens overnight. It happens in the quiet work of doing the morning ritual, eating the balanced meals, taking the walks, responding to cravings with grace, and returning gently after the hard days. It happens in the accumulated evidence that you are showing up for yourself, again and again, until you cannot deny it anymore.

You are becoming her already. If you have made it this far in this book, you are already doing the work. You are already the woman who is rebuilding. You are already reclaiming something that was never really lost, just hidden for a while.

In the next chapter, we are going to talk about what to actually put on your plate, in practical detail. The foods that support your body, your hormones, your energy, and your calm. The foods that love you back. Turn the page when you are ready, and let's get into the delicious part of this journey.

7

THE 21-DAY PINK SALT RESET PLAN

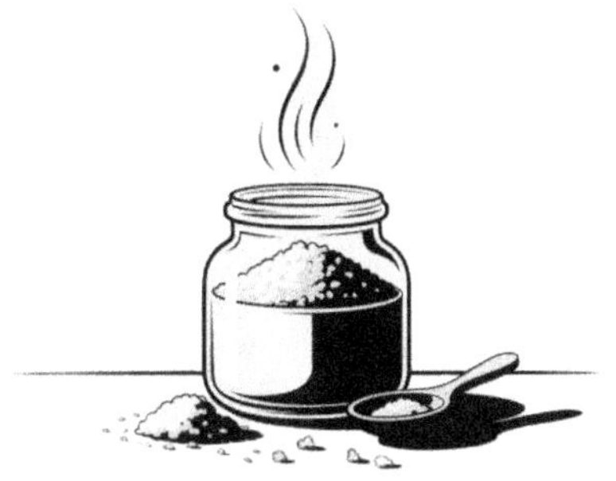

YOU HAVE SPENT FIVE CHAPTERS BUILDING UNDERSTANDING.

You know why your body has changed, and you know it is not your fault. You know what the morning ritual is, why it works, and how to make it automatic. You know the real causes of your bloating and the practical strategies that address them. You know why your cravings are not a character flaw and how to build meals that reduce them. You know what is stealing your energy and how to get it back.

Now it is time to put all of it together into something you can actually do — day by day, in your real life, starting from wherever you are right now.

This is the 21-Day Pink Salt Reset. Not a punishment, not a perfect protocol, not a program that requires you to become a different person before you can begin. It is a structured, compassionate, practical framework designed to take everything you have learned and translate it into twenty-one days of consistent action — action that will produce real, feelable results and lay the foundation for a way of living that continues long after the final day.

WHY 21 DAYS MATTERS

There is something important about a defined timeframe that open-ended intentions cannot replicate.

When a wellness goal has no clear structure — just "I want to eat better" or "I want to lose weight" — the mind has nowhere specific to put its energy. Every day is simultaneously a fresh start and an undefined stretch of effort with no visible endpoint. This ambiguity is one of the most reliable routes to inconsistency, because the brain functions better with clear, bounded tasks than with perpetual, shapeless commitments.

Twenty-one days is long enough to create genuine, measurable change. It is long enough for morning habits to become automatic, for the gut to begin responding to improved food choices, for sleep patterns to shift, for the body's inflammation and water retention to settle, and for the neurological grooves of new behavior to deepen into something that begins to feel natural. Research on habit formation consistently shows that three weeks of consistent practice — not perfect practice, but consistent — is sufficient to begin the transition from deliberate effort to something closer to automatic behavior.

Twenty-one days is also short enough to feel genuinely achievable. Not a six-month overhaul. Not a lifetime commitment made on a Monday morning when motivation is high but which collapses under the inevitable pressures of real life by the following weekend. Just twenty-one days. You can see the other end of it. You can hold the whole thing in your mind as a single, completable task. That bounded quality creates a different relationship with commitment — one that is specific, energizing, and psychologically manageable.

And twenty-one days, practiced with the strategies in this book, will produce changes you can feel. Not dramatic before-and-after transformation — this book has been honest with you throughout, and it will not start over-promising here. But real changes: a midsection that feels less tight and uncomfortable, mornings that begin with more clarity and less heaviness, afternoons with a different quality of energy, fewer of the urgent cravings that used to derail your evenings, and — perhaps most importantly — a rebuilt sense of trust in your own ability to care for yourself consistently.

That last change is the most significant of all, because it is the one that makes everything else possible long after the twenty-one days are over.

This is a reset, not a sentence. Let's begin.

HOW TO USE THIS PLAN

Before we walk through the three weeks in detail, a few important principles for using this plan in the way that will serve you best.

Follow it imperfectly rather than abandon it perfectly. The greatest enemy of a twenty-one-day plan is the all-or-nothing thinking that declares any imperfection a failure requiring a restart. The woman who follows this plan at seventy or eighty percent consistency for twenty-one consecutive days will produce far more lasting change than the woman who follows it perfectly for six days, experiences one difficult day, and decides she needs to start again from day one. Imperfect progress, kept in motion, is the whole strategy.

Adapt it to your life. This plan is built on principles that work, but the specific expression of those principles in your day will look different from anyone else's. If a suggested meal time does not work with your schedule, adjust it. If the evening walk is not possible on certain days, do it at lunch instead. If one week is particularly stressful, simplify rather than quit. The plan is a framework, not a rulebook, and you are intelligent enough to apply its spirit to the particular circumstances of your life.

Measure progress in multiple currencies. The scale is one measure of one thing. It is not the whole story of your progress, and treating it as such will distort your experience of these twenty-one days in ways that are neither accurate nor helpful. We will talk in detail about the full range of progress markers later in this chapter. For now, simply begin with the intention to notice more than the number.

You do not have to be ready. You do not have to have the perfect week ahead, the perfectly stocked kitchen, the completely clear schedule. These conditions will never all exist simultaneously, and waiting for them is how weeks become months and months become years. You begin from wherever you are. Today, if possible. Tomorrow morning at the latest.

WEEK ONE: REDUCE BLOAT AND BUILD MOMENTUM

The first week of the reset has one primary purpose: to establish the morning ritual as a daily anchor and to make the dietary and lifestyle changes most likely to produce the visible, feelable results that build momentum for everything that follows.

The focus of week one is simple and deliberately modest. You are not attempting to overhaul everything simultaneously. You are making three to four specific, targeted changes that address the most common drivers of bloating, energy depletion, and digestive discomfort — and you are practicing them consistently for seven days.

Every morning of week one begins the same way. Before your coffee, before your phone, before any of the day's demands arrive — your pink salt morning ritual. Warm water, a pinch of pink salt, the optional squeeze of lemon, the few quiet minutes of intentional beginning. If you have been practicing this ritual since Chapter 3, week one is about deepening its consistency. If you are beginning today, week one is where the practice takes root.

Hydration beyond the morning ritual is the second focus of week one. Aim for six to eight glasses of water distributed across the day, with particular attention to drinking water before each meal and in the mid-afternoon window when dehydration most often passes itself off as hunger and fatigue. Keep a glass or bottle visible and accessible throughout the day. Remove the friction. If plain water feels tedious, add a slice of lemon or cucumber, or drink herbal teas to supplement your intake.

Meals during week one are built on one simple principle: reduce the processed, increase the whole. You are not following a specific calorie target or eliminating any particular food group. You are simply shifting the composition of your eating toward more meals assembled from recognizable, unprocessed ingredients, and away from the packaged and convenience foods that carry the hidden sodium, artificial additives, and fermentable compounds that drive so much of the bloating and digestive discomfort you are trying to resolve.

This does not mean every meal needs to be cooked from scratch. It means a lunch of grilled chicken and a salad rather than a packaged sandwich. Eggs and vegetables for breakfast rather than cereal. Dinner built around a protein source with vegetables rather than a ready meal. Simple, accessible shifts that require modest planning but not excessive time or culinary skill.

Meal timing matters in week one, particularly the evening meal. Aim to finish eating at least two hours before bed, and keep the evening meal lighter than your lunch. This single change — eating less, and earlier, in the evenings — produces noticeable improvements in morning comfort for many women within the first three to four days.

After at least one meal each day, take a ten-to-fifteen-minute walk. It does not need to be brisk or structured as exercise. It is a digestive walk — a gentle physical activation that supports gut motility, reduces post-meal blood sugar peaks, and helps gas move through the digestive system before you settle back into sitting. Many women find this the most immediately impactful change of the entire first week, producing a noticeably less bloated evening and a flatter, more comfortable morning.

By the end of week one, notice what has shifted. Many women report feeling less tight and uncomfortable by evening. Morning puffiness often reduces. Digestion may feel more regular and less unpredictable. The morning ritual will have been completed seven times — and that track record, however modest, is the first real evidence that you are someone who does this. That evidence matters more than the scale.

If the scale has moved, that is encouraging. If it has not moved yet, or has moved in ways that seem counterintuitive, remember that week one changes are often primarily driven by reductions in water retention and digestive gas — changes that show up as comfort and physical ease before they show up as weight loss. You are building the foundation. The foundation always comes first.

WEEK TWO: STABILIZE ENERGY AND REDUCE CRAVINGS

Week two builds directly on the momentum of week one. The morning ritual is becoming more automatic. The reduced processed food intake is beginning to shift the inflammatory load that drove some of your bloating. The daily walks are becoming part of your rhythm.

Now the focus shifts to the fuel that powers your day — specifically, to the meal composition and daily habits that stabilize blood sugar, reduce craving intensity, and create the kind of sustained energy that makes the second half of every day feel fundamentally different from the crash-and-reach pattern that many women have been living with for years.

Protein becomes the conscious priority of week two. At every meal — not occasionally, not when it is convenient, but at every meal — include a deliberate, meaningful source of protein. Eggs, Greek yogurt, cottage cheese, lean meat, fish, legumes, tofu. The specific sources matter far less than the consistency. A breakfast with twenty to thirty grams of protein sets a blood sugar and satiety tone that carries you to lunch without the mid-morning cravings that derail so many good intentions before noon. A lunch with adequate protein means an afternoon that does not crater at three o'clock. A dinner with sufficient protein supports overnight tissue repair and reduces the morning hunger that can lead to poor breakfast choices.

If you currently eat breakfasts that are primarily carbohydrate-based — cereal, toast, fruit, granola — this is the week to experiment with protein-forward alternatives. Scrambled eggs with vegetables. Greek yogurt with berries and a small handful of nuts. A smoothie that includes protein powder, nut butter, or Greek yogurt rather than consisting primarily of fruit and juice. The shift in how you feel through the morning will be noticeable within a few days, and it is one of the most convincing demonstrations that food composition matters as much as food quantity.

Sleep becomes an explicit focus in week two. Not because it was unimportant in week one, but because one week of improved eating and hydration often creates enough physiological stability to make sleep improvements more accessible. Choose a consistent bedtime and wake time and maintain them across the week, including weekends as closely as practical. Create a genuine wind-down routine for the thirty to sixty minutes before bed — screens off or significantly reduced, lighting dimmed, something genuinely relaxing that allows the nervous system to downshift before you ask it to sleep. The bedroom should be cool, dark, and quiet.

If night waking or early waking is a significant issue for you — which is very common during perimenopause and menopause — week two is the time to begin addressing it directly. Avoiding alcohol in the evenings, eating your last meal at least two to three hours before bed, limiting caffeine after midday, and establishing the wind-down routine are all first-line strategies that produce meaningful improvement for many women without requiring any medical intervention.

Stress resets are the third new addition of week two. These are brief, intentional interruptions to the stress accumulation that happens throughout the day — not elaborate practices, but small physiological pivots that prevent cortisol from building to the level where it drives afternoon cravings and evening emotional eating. A minute of slow, deliberate breathing before a stressful meeting. A five-minute walk at midday that has nothing to do with exercise and everything to do with breaking the continuous cognitive demand cycle. A conscious pause between finishing work and beginning the evening — a transition ritual that signals to your nervous system that one part of the day is over and a different quality of time is beginning.

These micro-resets do not eliminate stress. They interrupt its accumulation in ways that prevent it from reaching the craving-driving, sleep-disrupting, belly-fat-promoting levels that make midlife health management so much harder than it needs to be.

By the end of week two, the changes become more integrated and more felt. Energy through the day typically stabilizes in ways that are genuinely noticeable — not dramatic, not the sudden abundant vitality of fantasy, but a steadiness that replaces the rollercoaster. Cravings, for many women, begin to feel more like mild preferences than urgent demands. Sleep, when the week two strategies are practiced consistently, often shows meaningful improvement in depth or continuity. The morning ritual is fourteen days old, and it feels — perhaps for the first time — genuinely like yours.

WEEK THREE: BUILD LASTING WEIGHT-LOSS HABITS

The third week is where the reset becomes a foundation rather than a program — where the practices of the first two weeks, now established with some consistency, begin to settle into the fabric of how you live rather than feeling like something you are doing on top of your life.

The focus of week three is sustainability, identity, and the gradual expansion of the habits you have built into a way of caring for yourself that you can genuinely imagine continuing indefinitely.

Movement receives more intentional attention in week three. The daily walks from week one are, by now, a natural part of your routine. Week three invites a small expansion — not a dramatic new exercise commitment, but a gentle step toward incorporating some resistance-based movement into your week. Two sessions of twenty to thirty minutes, using whatever format is accessible to you: a simple bodyweight routine at home, a set of resistance bands, a gym visit, a beginner strength class. The goal is not performance or perfection. It is introducing the stimulus for muscle maintenance that becomes increasingly important for metabolic health after forty, and doing so in a way that feels manageable and sustainable rather than overwhelming.

Flexible mindset is perhaps the most important skill to consciously develop in week three. By this point, you have likely had at least one or two days that did not go according to plan — a missed morning ritual, an evening of emotional eating, a day of travel or illness or family crisis that disrupted the routine. The way you handled those interruptions — whether you returned immediately and without drama, or whether you allowed them to spiral into extended derailment — has been teaching you something about your current relationship with imperfection.

Week three is the time to practice returning. Not from a dramatic failure, but from the minor disruptions that real life consistently delivers. The skill of returning — quietly, without excessive self-examination, without theatrical recommitment — is the single most important long-term habit skill you can develop. It is more valuable than any specific food choice or exercise routine, because it is the skill that makes all other skills sustainable across the months and years of real life.

Eating in week three continues and deepens the patterns established in weeks one and two, with a new dimension: planning. Not rigid meal planning with every ingredient mapped out, but the kind of light-touch planning that prevents the reactive, poor-quality food choices that happen when hunger arrives and nothing prepared is available. Knowing what you will eat for dinner before three o'clock in the afternoon. Having protein-rich breakfasts stocked in the refrigerator. Keeping a few simple, nourishing snacks accessible for the moments between meals when hunger bridges are needed. This level of planning requires perhaps twenty minutes at the start of the week and prevents dozens of impulsive food decisions that the depleted, hungry, end-of-day brain is not well-equipped to make wisely.

The identity shift of week three is subtle but significant. You have been doing this for seventeen, eighteen, nineteen days. You are not someone trying to establish a morning ritual — you are someone who has a morning ritual. You are not trying to eat more protein — you are someone who builds protein into your meals as a matter of course. You are not trying to walk daily — you are a woman who moves her body every day. These distinctions, small as they sound, create a different internal relationship with the behaviors. They shift from things you are effortfully doing to things that are simply true of you. And that shift in identity is the foundation upon which lasting change is built.

On the final days of week three, spend a few minutes thinking forward rather than only backward. Not to judge or assess what you have not yet achieved, but to plan what comes next — how you will carry the morning ritual, the protein-forward eating, the daily movement, and the stress management practices beyond day twenty-one into the days and weeks that follow. Because the reset is designed to produce change that outlasts its twenty-one days, and the choices you make on day twenty-two will determine whether what you have built continues to grow.

WHAT TO TRACK BEYOND THE SCALE

The scale is a single instrument measuring a single variable, and that variable — total body weight — includes muscle, fat, bone, water, and the contents of your digestive tract at any given moment. As a daily tracker of progress during a hormonal reset designed for women over forty, it is among the least informative tools available to you, and relying on it as the primary measure of whether this is working will consistently provide a distorted picture.

Here is what to track instead — or alongside, if you choose to weigh yourself at all.

Bloating and digestive comfort, observed morning and evening. Is your abdomen less tight when you wake up? Does the evening distension that was constant a few weeks ago arrive less reliably, or feel less pronounced when it does? These changes often precede scale movement and are a direct measure of the gut-level improvements the reset is designed to produce.

Energy quality, particularly in the afternoon. Does the three o'clock crash arrive with the same force it did before week one? Are you reaching the end of a working day with something resembling functional energy rather than running on empty? Energy improvements often appear in the second week and deepen progressively.

Sleep quality, including ease of falling asleep, number of nighttime wakings, and how rested you feel in the morning. For many women, sleep improvements are among the most emotionally significant changes of the entire reset, because the cumulative effects of poor sleep are so pervasive and so undermining of every other aspect of wellbeing.

Mood and emotional steadiness. The hormonal stabilization that comes from better sleep, more consistent blood sugar, and reduced inflammatory load often produces mood improvements that women describe as feeling more like themselves — less reactive, less anxious, less prone to the emotional swings that perimenopause can intensify. This is not always visible to the outside world, but it is deeply felt from the inside.

Craving intensity and frequency. Are the three o'clock sugar urges as urgent as they were? Is the evening kitchen pull less insistent? The progression from cravings that feel unmanageable to cravings that feel like mild preferences is a meaningful sign of blood sugar and hormonal stabilization.

How your clothes feel. Not a specific size, not a measurement — simply whether the clothes you are wearing day to day feel more comfortable, less confining, more accurately representative of the body you are actually living in. For many women, this is the most satisfying and reliable marker of genuine change.

Consistency itself. How many of the twenty-one mornings have included the ritual? How many evenings have ended with a ten-minute walk after dinner? How many days have included protein at every meal? Consistency is progress, regardless of what the scale reports, because consistent behavior is what produces lasting physiological change.

IF PROGRESS FEELS SLOW

There will be some women reading this who reach week two or three of the reset and feel that the changes are not arriving quickly enough, or that their body is responding differently from the experiences described in these pages. This section is for you.

Slow progress is still progress. It is also the most common kind for women navigating perimenopause and menopause, because the hormonal context of this life stage genuinely does make the body's rate of change more variable than it was in earlier decades. What took two weeks at thirty may take six weeks at forty-five. This is not failure. It is physiology — and the same physiology that makes change feel slower also makes consistent, sustained effort more important and more permanently transformative.

Bodies are different. This cannot be said often enough in a wellness culture that tends to present singular, universal experiences of what a protocol should produce and how quickly. Your gut microbiome, your hormonal timeline, your sleep history, your stress load, your thyroid function, your activity history — all of these create an individual context for this reset that cannot be compared to anyone else's. The woman who loses four pounds in the first two weeks and the woman who feels lighter without any scale change are both potentially experiencing exactly the right response from their particular body.

Internal healing is often invisible before it is visible. The reduction in gut inflammation, the improvement in insulin sensitivity, the shift in gut microbiome composition, the beginning of circadian rhythm regulation — these changes happen before they show up in the mirror or on the scale. They are happening regardless of what any external measure tells you. Trust the process enough to let it complete.

If progress genuinely feels stalled after the full twenty-one days, the gentlest first adjustment is not to add more restriction but to examine the fundamentals: Is sleep adequately prioritized? Is protein consistently sufficient? Is hydration genuinely consistent throughout the day? Is stress chronically elevated in ways that are overriding the other efforts? Most of the time, the answer to slow progress lives in one of these areas rather than in the need for a more extreme approach.

WHAT HAPPENS AFTER DAY 21

Day twenty-one is not a finish line. It is a milestone on a longer journey, and how you treat it will determine whether the twenty-one days become the beginning of a lasting shift or a period of good habits that gradually dissolve when the structure ends.

The simplest and most powerful thing you can do on day twenty-two is the same thing you did on day one: make your morning ritual water and drink it before your coffee.

From that anchor, everything else extends naturally. The eating patterns of the reset are not a temporary diet to be abandoned but a way of feeding yourself that simply works better for your body at this stage of life. The daily movement is not a program with an end date but a permanent feature of a life that includes consistent physical activation. The sleep practices are not a twenty-one-day experiment but the ongoing investment in recovery that your body genuinely requires.

If you want more structure, repeat the reset. Many women find that cycling through the twenty-one days two or three times, with the growing confidence and competence of repetition, produces progressively deeper results. The second round is easier than the first. The third round begins to feel like simply living.

If you are ready to expand, consider adding strength training as a more central feature of your weekly movement rather than the modest resistance work introduced in week three. Two to three sessions per week of progressive resistance exercise — gradually increasing the challenge as your strength improves — is the single most impactful long-term intervention for metabolic health, body composition, and physical vitality for women over forty. It does not need to be complicated or expensive, and the results over months and years are genuinely transformative.

Continue building on what worked. Notice which elements of the reset produced the most significant changes for you — was it the sleep improvements? The protein-forward meals? The daily walks? The morning ritual? These are your high-leverage habits, the ones that produce outsized returns for you specifically. Double down on maintaining them before adding anything new.

Set a new focus. Perhaps the next phase is more intentional strength building. Perhaps it is deepening your stress management practices. Perhaps it is exploring specific dietary adjustments — reducing alcohol, addressing a particular food sensitivity, improving the quality of your carbohydrate sources. The reset has given you a foundation of consistency and self-knowledge from which any of these directions can be pursued with confidence rather than desperation.

YOUR FRESH START BEGINS NOW

Somewhere in these pages, you recognized yourself.

You recognized the frustration of a body that seemed to change its rules overnight. You recognized the bloating that arrives by evening and refuses to explain itself. You recognized the exhaustion that coffee barely touches and the cravings that arrive with the force of an instruction rather than a suggestion. You recognized the starting over, and the self-doubt, and the quiet wondering whether you are simply someone who cannot manage this.

You are not that person. You never were.

You are a woman in the middle of a significant biological transition, armed with better information than you had before you opened this book, equipped with practical tools that are grounded in reality rather than fantasy, and capable of exactly the kind of consistent, compassionate self-care that produces the changes you are looking for.

The morning ritual is ready. The warm water and the pinch of pink salt and the quiet few minutes before the day begins — these are yours now. Not a miracle, not a gimmick, but a daily act of intention that signals to your body and your brain that today begins differently. That you are someone who does this. That this day, and all the choices that follow from it, belong to a woman who takes care of herself.

Twenty-one days is all you are committing to right now. Not a lifetime of perfection. Not an idealized future version of yourself that requires everything to change simultaneously. Just twenty-one mornings of ritual, twenty-one days of consistent nourishment, twenty-one opportunities to practice returning to yourself after the inevitable disruptions that real life delivers.

You do not need to be ready. You do not need ideal conditions. You do not need to resolve the self-doubt before you begin, because the self-doubt dissolves in the doing — replaced, day by day, with the quiet, unshakeable evidence of a woman who keeps her promises to herself.

The woman you want to be is not ahead of you somewhere in the future, waiting on the other side of a transformation. She is here, now, choosing to begin.

The water is warm. The salt is ready. The morning is yours.

Begin.

CONCLUSION: YOUR NEW CHAPTER STARTS NOW

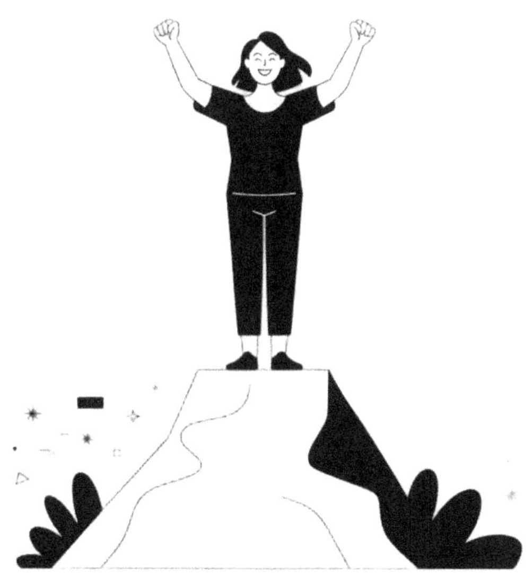

YOU MADE IT HERE.

Not to an ending to a beginning. And there is a significant difference between those two things that is worth pausing to acknowledge before we close.

When you first picked up this book, you were carrying something. Perhaps it was frustration — the particular kind that comes from trying genuinely hard and not seeing the results that effort should produce. Perhaps it was confusion about a body that seemed to have renegotiated its terms without your input. Perhaps it was a quiet, accumulated exhaustion from the years of starting over, of Monday resolutions and Thursday setbacks, of looking in the mirror and not quite recognizing the woman looking back.

Whatever you were carrying when you arrived here, something has shifted. Not because these pages performed magic — this book made you a promise early on that it would not deal in magic, and it has kept that promise. But because understanding changes things. Because knowing why your body is behaving the way it is replaces the shame of personal failure with the clarity of biological reality. Because having tools that actually work for the body you are living in now — not the body you had at thirty-two, not an idealized body in optimal circumstances, but yours, now, in the complexity of this particular life and this particular stage — changes what is possible.

You are not the same reader who opened Chapter 1. Take a moment to recognize that.

CELEBRATE HOW FAR YOU HAVE COME

Look at what you actually know now that you did not know before.

You understand that the hormonal shifts of perimenopause and menopause are real, significant, and responsible for a wide range of the changes that have felt so disorienting — the belly fat that accumulates differently, the sleep that no longer restores the way it once did, the cravings that arrive with a force that has nothing to do with weakness and everything to do with neurochemistry. You know that estrogen and progesterone and cortisol and insulin are not abstract scientific terms but active players in how you feel every single day, and that supporting them with the right conditions produces real, felt results.

You understand that bloating is not the same as fat gain, that the scale measures far more than progress, and that the morning puffiness and evening tightness that used to feel like permanent features of your body are dynamic, responsive, and significantly within your influence. You have practical strategies for addressing them that are grounded in how your body actually works rather than in the wishful thinking of quick-fix culture.

You understand why restrictive diets have failed you, and you have released the self-blame that those failures used to generate. You know that the problem was never your willpower. It was the approach — a strategy designed for a different hormonal environment, applied with determination and good faith to a body that needed something different.

You have a morning ritual. A small, consistent, daily act of intention that begins each day with care rather than chaos, that anchors your hydration and your mindset before the demands of the world arrive, and that has been proven — in your own experience, if you have been practicing it — to change the quality of everything that follows.

You have a 21-day framework that translates understanding into action, that provides the structure your motivated self designed for the inevitable days when motivation is nowhere to be found, and that has already begun producing the kind of changes that matter most: not dramatic, not overnight, but real, felt, and sustainable.

This is not nothing. This is genuinely, meaningfully something. Own it.

THIS WAS NEVER ABOUT PERFECTION

Here is what real change looks like, and it is important that you hold onto this picture in the weeks and months ahead.

It does not look like an unbroken streak of perfect days. It does not look like a diet followed with complete compliance, or a morning ritual completed every single morning without exception, or a body that responds on schedule with predictable, linear improvement. It does not look like the before-and-after photographs of wellness marketing, where the transformation is total and the expression in the after photo suggests that all previous difficulty has been permanently resolved.

Real change looks like mostly. Like often. Like getting back to it on Thursday after a difficult Tuesday and Wednesday. It looks like a morning ritual completed on the tired days as well as the energized ones. It looks like a meal plan followed imperfectly across a week that contained an unexpected work crisis, a sick child, and a dinner out that went further off-plan than intended — and then continued anyway, because the imperfect week was not a failure requiring restart but simply a week, one of many, in a life where consistency matters more than any individual day.

The pressure to be perfect is one of the most reliably destructive forces in women's wellness, and it operates so subtly and so pervasively that many women do not even notice it governing their choices until they have already declared themselves failed for the forty-seventh time. Releasing that pressure is not lowering your standards. It is meeting your actual life with an approach that can survive contact with it.

You are allowed to be imperfect at this. In fact, you must be imperfect at this, because there is no other way to do it that lasts.

Progress is not a straight line. It is an uneven, sometimes confusing, occasionally frustrating series of forward movements and minor setbacks that, viewed over enough time, trends unambiguously in a direction you can feel. Keep the long view. A single difficult day changes nothing. A week of difficult days changes nothing that one genuinely good week cannot restore. You are never as far back as a discouraging moment makes you feel.

THE WINS BEYOND WEIGHT LOSS

Before we talk about what comes next, take a moment to inventory the changes that may not show up on a scale but that matter enormously to the quality of your daily life.

Your mornings. Are they different from the mornings you were waking up to before this reset? Is there a quality of intention in them that was not there before — even a small one, even on the hard days? The few minutes of quiet ritual before the day begins represent something larger than hydration. They represent a daily choice to begin by caring for yourself, and that choice, made consistently, gradually reshapes the relationship you have with your own well-being in ways that extend far beyond any single habit.

Your relationship with food. Is it slightly less fraught? Are there moments when you make a food choice from genuine nourishment and desire rather than from urgency and then regret? Are there evenings when the craving arrives and you respond to it with curiosity rather than catastrophe — pausing, hydrating, asking what you actually need, making a considered choice? These moments are evidence of a fundamentally different relationship developing, and they deserve to be recognized.

Your energy. Are there hours in your day that feel different than they did six weeks ago — more available, less dependent on caffeine, less subject to the dramatic mid-afternoon cliff? The woman whose energy has shifted from rollercoaster to something steadier has not simply lost weight. She has changed the metabolic and hormonal architecture of her daily experience. That is significant.

Your sleep. If the wind-down practices and the eating changes have improved the quality of your nights — even modestly, even partially — the downstream effects of that improvement touch everything: mood, cravings, energy, patience, cognitive clarity, emotional resilience, the ease of every other healthy choice. Sleep is not a passive absence of wakefulness. It is the foundation on which everything else is built, and any improvement in it is worth celebrating explicitly.

Your confidence. Not just in how you look, though that matters and is real, but in how you feel about your ability to care for yourself. The quiet, gradually accumulating evidence that you are a woman who keeps her promises to herself, who gets back to her practices after disruption, who has a morning ritual and a daily walk and a way of eating that supports rather than undermines her health — this confidence is deeper and more durable than any number on any scale.

These are the wins that last. These are the changes that compound over months and years into a fundamentally different quality of life.

WHAT TO DO NEXT

The most important thing you can do the morning after you finish this book is exactly what you have been doing every morning since you began: make your ritual water, find your few minutes of quiet, and begin the day with intention.

Everything else extends from that foundation.

If the 21-day reset is complete, consider repeating it. The second round will be easier than the first — the habits will require less conscious effort, the results will build on the foundation already laid, and the confidence of having done it once will change the quality of your engagement with doing it again. Many women find that two or three cycles of the reset produce progressively deeper integration of the practices into their ordinary life, until the reset and their ordinary life become indistinguishable from each other.

If you are ready to add strength training as a more central feature of your movement, begin simply and begin consistently. Two sessions per week of resistance-based movement — bodyweight exercises, resistance bands, weights, whatever format is accessible and sustainable for your life — produces meaningful metabolic and body composition benefits for women over forty that cardio alone cannot match. Start where you are, progress gradually, and prioritize consistency over intensity.

Continue protecting sleep as though it is the most important wellness practice you have, because for women navigating hormonal transition, it almost certainly is. The wind-down routine, the consistent sleep and wake times, the reduction of sleep-disrupting habits in the evening — these are not temporary interventions for the duration of a program. They are permanent features of a life that takes your recovery and restoration seriously.

Keep learning your body. The self-knowledge you have developed through this reset — the awareness of what your body responds to, where your personal triggers lie, which habits produce the most noticeable positive changes for you specifically — is more valuable than any external protocol. You are the expert on your own experience. Trust what you have observed, and continue refining your approach based on what genuinely works rather than what works for someone else.

WHEN MOTIVATION DROPS

It will. This is not pessimism. It is the honest acknowledgment of how motivation actually works.

Motivation is a wave, not a tide. It rises and it falls, and the falling is not evidence that you do not care or do not want this enough. It is evidence that you are a human being operating in a life that contains difficulty, fatigue, competing demands, and seasons of genuine hardship alongside its joys. Expecting sustained, consistent motivation is expecting something that no person experiences, regardless of how committed or successful they appear.

What carries you through the inevitable low-motivation periods is not a renewed determination to feel motivated. It is the routines and habits and environmental designs that make your healthy practices automatic enough to happen even when the feeling of wanting to do them is absent.

This is why the morning ritual matters so much. Not on the mornings when you feel energized and hopeful and certain that today will be a good day — doing it then is easy and requires nothing from you. It matters on the Tuesday when you slept badly and the week is already overwhelming before it has properly started and the last thing in the world you feel like doing is being intentional. On that morning, the ritual is the thing that carries you. Not because it is magical, but because it is automatic enough now that you do it before your unmotivated mind has had a chance to talk you out of it. And having done it, you have made one good choice. And one good choice makes a second slightly more likely. And the day that started with dread ends with a quiet sense of having managed.

You are never back at zero. Not after a difficult week, not after a missed month, not after a period of genuine life disruption that pushed every wellness practice to the background. The understanding you have built does not disappear. The body-awareness you have developed does not reset. The self-knowledge you have accumulated is yours, permanently. Every restart is not a return to the beginning — it is a continuation from a more informed, more capable, more self-aware place than the time before.

Restart quickly. Without ceremony. Without the weight of what was missed. Simply return to the morning ritual and continue.

BECOMING THE WOMAN YOU TRUST AGAIN

There is a version of you that this entire book has been in service of — not a different person, not a younger person, not a version of you requiring a different body or a different history. The same you, living in this body, in this life, at this age, with this accumulated wisdom and this particular combination of strength and softness. That version of you simply trusts herself.

She trusts that she will do her morning ritual because she has done it enough times that it has become part of her identity. She trusts that when a craving arrives with force, she has a response ready that does not involve shame or surrender. She trusts that a difficult day will not become a derailed week, because she has practiced returning too many times to believe the story that imperfection means failure.

She trusts her body — not to be perfect, not to respond on any predetermined schedule, but to be genuinely responsive to consistent care. She has seen it. The morning she woke up and her midsection felt different. The afternoon the crash did not arrive. The evening she made a food choice from genuine hunger and genuine satisfaction and felt neither guilty nor virtuous about it — just fed. She has evidence now. Not from someone else's experience, not from before-and-after photographs of strangers, but from her own body, responding to her own consistent care.

This trust is what changes everything. Not the information, not the plan, not the specific habits — though all of those matter. The trust. Because a woman who trusts herself makes different choices on the hard days. She returns more quickly after disruption. She extends herself more compassion when she falls short and more credit when she succeeds. She approaches the ongoing project of her own health not as a series of attempts separated by failures, but as a continuous practice — imperfect, evolving, genuinely hers.

That woman is who you have been becoming through these pages. She is not ahead of you in some imagined future. She is emerging from the choices you have already made — the mornings you showed up for your ritual, the meals you built with intention, the days you walked after dinner, the moments you paused before a craving and asked what you actually needed.

She is here. She has been here all along, waiting for the right conditions to become fully visible.

A FINAL WORD

You deserve to feel well in your body.

Not as a reward for achieving a certain size or weight. Not contingent on a month of perfect choices or a scale number that meets some external standard. Now. As a woman who is navigating one of the most significant biological transitions of her life with courage and curiosity and the willingness to learn and try and try again.

The pink salt morning ritual is a small thing. A glass of warm water, a pinch of mineral salt, a few quiet minutes before the day begins. It will not transform your hormones or erase the effects of menopause or solve everything at once. It was never designed to.

What it will do — what it has been designed to do — is give you a starting point. A daily anchor. A small, consistent, morning act of self-care that says: today, I begin by giving my body something it needs. And from that beginning, with the understanding and tools this book has given you, everything else becomes a little more possible.

The water is warm. The salt is ready. The morning is yours — this one, and the one after, and all the ones that follow.

You know what to do now.

Go and do it beautifully.

www.ingramcontent.com/pod-product-compliance
Lightning Source LLC
Chambersburg PA
CBHW051813050726
47598CB00006B/2537